Best wishes,

Anne

ITALY ON MY MIND

Anne Brewer

MINERVA PRESS
LONDON
MONTREUX   LOS ANGELES   SYDNEY

ITALY ON MY MIND
Copyright © Anne Brewer 1997

ISBN 1 86106 550 7

First Published 1997 by
MINERVA PRESS
195 Knightsbridge
London SW7 1RE

Printed in Great Britain for Minerva Press

ITALY ON MY MIND

In memory of Linda
With grateful thanks to my mother, Ady and Philip for
their help and support.

Contents

Chapter One

January 1990

I opened my eyes wearily, ignoring the dull, lingering ache in my muscles, and looked very slowly around the room. It was fairly dark, as the curtains were still tightly drawn. I didn't have the strength to go and open them. The light was filtering gently in, dappled green – taking on the texture of the curtains. A forest glade, where you could lie stiffly on a firm, comfortable bed and despite your overwhelmingly muggy thoughts, be conduced to day-dream!

I was thirty-three and *ill*, in England, at home with my parents. My mind just couldn't get used to the idea, and was continually reaching for the place I'd left behind, Conegliano, Veneto, in Italy, which I'd departed from such a short time ago, when I'd flown home to my parents, for the long-awaited Christmas holiday.

I'd had severe pneumonia start on Christmas Day, and now the influenza that had overwhelmed me would not lift. Only my thoughts could move around freely, as my limbs were almost entirely bed-bound.

In Conegliano, Veneto, I fondly thought, I had my small, but comfortable, and dare I call it, even somewhat stylish flat. It was on the second floor, behind a glass front door surrounded by cork-tiled walls. As I lay in silence, alone in my room in Ridlow, I reflected that those Italian cork tiles absorbed the clip-clop of all the heels, including the metal-tipped ones, and made the stairways and corridors – well, not quite cosy – but certainly extremely friendly and never impersonal or cold. The hollow echoing voices of hospital stairs and corridors that I had known in other times were never there. Voices were tempered and interesting, not disembodied, alienating, or seal-like. They made you want to open your front door and listen in avidly to other people's conversations! Even if I was there, I reflected sadly,

I wouldn't be able to rush out and talk to anyone, for my legs wouldn't carry me!

The earth-coloured terracotta tiles and white painted walls in Conegliano always reminded me of sunshine and of sitting inside, warmed through but feeling fresh, during the hottest part of lingering summer days. Not like England, where in our house in Ridlow wall-to-wall carpeting seemed one of the best ways of combating the cooler, damper climate. I looked at it and it comforted me in a different way – it didn't remind me of sunshine, but of cosiness, and of sitting on the warm floor cuddled up by the fire or a glowing radiator, with a favourite book. I preferred plain-coloured carpets, where, as with the terracotta tiles, you wouldn't have a mass of brown or blue swirls in which anything could hide, but where every object placed upon them would stand out clearly.

That little scorpion I'd come home to once after work in Italy! A friend had that year very kindly looked after my several pot plants over the summer, when I'd taken the school holidays in England. She'd given them back – with a scorpion inside – no doubt to keep the earwigs company which had crawled in too! How else could they ever have all arrived on my terracotta entrance hall on the *second* floor? The scorpion I disposed of by steeling myself and putting a small cooking basin over it, sliding a book underneath and quickly taking it downstairs to the shared garden and setting it free alongside the railway track. The earwigs soon followed suit!

Ah yes, there was no da-dum-di-dum, da-dum-di-dum noise heard from my bedroom in rural Ridlow – just as well, with the throbbing headaches that alternated with my muggy cotton wool thoughts, on and off throughout the days in bed. Those local and far-bound trains, that whooshed past in the night in Conegliano, certainly made themselves heard!   I smiled when I remembered the time my unsuspecting parents had stayed at my flat on holiday for a week, and my mother could not be dissuaded from believing that certain noisy and defiant trains might charge in through her bedroom window and flatten her when she opened it!

I looked up at the light in my bedroom in England – a white, conical, bobbled lampshade, with beige tassels hanging loosely down. It was not like the milky white chandelier that had been handcrafted like beautiful lilies stretching up and bending over and floating gently on the ceiling. My husband had insisted on it! I'd tried to persuade him to spend the money on a more practical, functional dishwasher. He'd been right though.

There was still no shadow of a contest for me now, as I lay there and thought about it. Glass, shaped and crafted, glistening and energising, had entered my consciousness when I lived in Venice, before moving to Conegliano, and I liked to believe that watching it sometimes had soothed tensions away, and allowed attainable dreams to form.

Every moulded contour of the unique chandelier that Umberto had insisted on had been studied and visually caressed by me thousands of times – whenever I'd had the time to lie in bed and pause awhile. It *was* functional after all – not only for the light! It was eminently peaceful.

In Conegliano, Veneto, my room was predominantly green and beige and wooden, just like my room at my parents'. My mother had kindly made up the light, floaty, simple curtains that allowed a similar green filtered light to pass through.

In both rooms there was peace, but perhaps in Italy the sense of that was a shade greater because of the fragile, yet strengthening glass light. And one further source: misty, greyish hues of Asolo, with a salmon sun about to set behind the mysterious hills. Asolo was a small, picturesque town nestling in those undulating hills, which I had visited many a Sunday afternoon. The painting, which also conjured up exciting fairy tales and adventures and dreams fulfilled, hung on my bedroom wall in Conegliano. I looked at it whenever I wanted to be spirited away somewhere! Yes, I'd bring those two peacemakers over to my bedroom in England, if I had to stay bed-bound in Ridlow. In the meantime, I'd do it in my mind. I was very lucky to have two such rooms.

I sipped the warm, reviving Paradise herbal tea that my mother had kindly brought me and, too tired to direct my mind in any specific direction, let my thoughts continue to meander lightly to where they could make me happier. I thought about going down impulsively in Conegliano to sit on the pale wooden seat in our communal garden below my flat, the bench just missing the cooling shadow of the small tree, and idly reading or relaxing in the sun. Oh, to be there now! I wished my temperature would go down. Invariably someone would leave their flat there and come down and have a short, but heartfelt chat, even bringing a coffee, and stop their busy routine for a refreshing breather.

At first I'd missed it, the privacy of our beautiful, secluded, peaceful garden at Ridlow, but gradually I'd adjusted to my new home and had joyfully gone down to the communal garden outside when I *was* in a sociable mood and ready for meeting people, thankful that there was such a place to go to! It didn't happen very often, unfortunately, for I was so busy, but whether I was in my flat in Italy or without, there I had never felt so lonely deep down inside as I did now.

My favourite month in Conegliano, I now realised, was mellow September, my birthday month. The centre of the town was decorated for the annual wine festival, later the chestnut festival and the 'Dama Castellana', a live chess game played on an open-air chessboard painted in the main square. Costumed opponents took part and the winners carried the lady of their dreams up to the castle afterwards.

Then, spontaneously, as I reminisced to myself, a feeling of severe weakness came over me, and at the same time, for some reason, my Italian bank, of all things, came vividly into my mind! I felt again those all-seeing eyes upon me – because I was English and word had soon got round – a combination of friendliness, warmth, curiosity and expertise, from the charming people who worked there.

One handsome young man in his early twenties would always fit in a quick chat over and beyond the call of duty, and I remembered he'd asked me out eventually! We'd gone to a house which stood halfway up the hillside, set back from the road, to meet his friends. We'd pushed a button to open the big wrought-iron gate to let the car in, and pushed a button to swing open the front door! We'd pushed a button to open the drinks cabinet, and pushed a button to slide back the television doors, to see a snatch of a comic chat show, while waiting for more young people to arrive. Then we'd all gone to a horrendously noisy disco and stood around without talking. It had slowly dawned on us how much difference a ten-year age gap could make in terms of interests. The enchantment with each other had gone. Without saying more, we'd gone our separate ways at the end of the night out. But it was fine. I was only slightly self-conscious going to the bank after that evening!

Ooh, now Roberto came into my mind too. Married and electrifying and so good-looking – who'd sent me a beautiful plant to say he'd always love me. My eight-year relationship with Umberto had been over for more than a year, when I'd met Roberto. I didn't know Dino then of course and would probably never have met him if Roberto and I had started something.

Dear Dino, after just about a year with kind-hearted, but forever busy Giovanni, Dino had become my boyfriend and, as I counted the days away from him now, I knew we had been together for a year and three months. He'd been lonely and, like me, had a broken marriage behind him. He'd been left as well. We shared a similar experience, although I had no children. He had a daughter, who stayed with her mum during the week and with him at weekends, so with that and his football matches on Sunday afternoons, I didn't see a great deal of him after Monday to Friday – but that was what he wanted – and we saw each other Sunday evenings and two or three times a week. We'd hit it off immediately, and had fun. When, I wondered, when would I get to see him again?

The day we'd gone to buy my new stereo system eased its way into my mind. I'd stipulated a small microphone too, so I could make recordings for my classes. Dino'd spent ages absorbedly weighing up all the many pros and cons of the systems available, until we'd finally decided on a Technics cassette player.

Whenever I'd had a little time after that, I'd pop on some lively music and practise my jazz dance steps for half an hour. Four nights a week I attended an excellent course. We danced to all types of music. We'd been working on the Latin American lambada up to Christmas. I'd come down with the severe recurring flu two days before we were due to perform the new routine in front of the public. I'd been heartbroken not to take part, as I'd worked so hard on learning the steps with all the home practice sessions and loved the music and the original choreography – I'd been too weak and ill even to go and watch the others perform.

As I lay disquietly in bed in Ridlow, I heard that lilting music dancing purposefully through my head and I already couldn't believe I'd done all those energetic combinations of steps, as all I could do now was make myself summon up the energy to stagger to the bathroom and back. I tried to think of incentives for rousing myself, but nothing worked. Terrible fatigue engulfed me, and I had never felt so weak for such a long period of time before. I somehow hadn't picked up after the pneumonia had ended. Wretched illness! What I really fancied was getting up and going for a tasty, freshly made pizza. That would be sure to get me going! When my family had come over to Conegliano for their last visit, we'd gone to Dino's and my favourite popular pizzeria. My other friends and I would go quite regularly too. At the end of English courses my students and I would go as a way of saying goodbye. Thanks to them I knew excellent places in Treviso and Venice, as well as Conegliano. In my mind, to feel less lonely, I tucked into a delicious pizza alla cipolla, as I munched my chicken sandwich!

It was so depressing feeling this rough – and not even being able to feebly talk to friends on the phone for more than a maximum of ten minutes, because, just as my thoughts were jumbled up, coherent words couldn't be extracted from my muddled head. I thanked God that at least I could cope with my memories!

I'd often wished I'd had more free time to socialise with my charming students, but commuting every weekday to Treviso and Venice and Mestre as I did, and living in Conegliano, meant a lot of to-ing and fro-ing. In general, I had to recharge my batteries closer to home and relax, see to running the house, and rest a bit at weekends.

But on the rare occasions my students and I did get together for weekend outings, the moments were to be treasured – as were the moments with close friends. A close-knit group from Venice University had organised a fun picnic with me on the pebbly banks of the meandering River Piave, not long ago, and in October, another lovely group had gone with me to the Sentiero dei Fiori, (Path of Flowers), in the mountains in Trentino.

I'd heard about the uplifting beauty of the mountains along the Sentiero dei Fiori for several busy months – from Max, whose home lay in Trentino. He was one of my lively, friendly, bright students at the University Linguistic Centre, studying diligently and well on a lower-intermediate English course. He told us at the warming-up session he wanted to become a teacher.

Manuela and Massimo, also studying at the Centro Linguistico Interfacolta, were keen to come, as were several others, who for one good reason or another were not able to manage it. We tried hard to find a suitable weekend we all had free and Max encouraged us again to stay Saturday *and* Sunday. But I simply and truly had too much laborious work on, with the computer exercises I was committed to writing for a book for Italian middle schools. So I had to make it a

Sunday, and we all decided to go for the day on October 7th. Little did I know it then, but it was to turn out to be just three months before I'd got this mysterious illness.

What lovely memories! Manuela and Massimo had met Riccardo and I punctually at the station in Conegliano and we'd all driven to the Trentino, where Max was expecting us. The car was full of anticipation, of joy, of laughter, of togetherness. The journey was spectacular and we duly arrived, light and ready for anything.

Giuseppe, Max's younger brother met us and we all went in and joined his parents for a hearty, cockle-warming lunch of beef stew and Trentino dumplings – with fresh fruit to follow. The meat seemed to taste different to other similar dishes I'd had in the past – there was a more pronounced, almost sweet and fruity flavour! Perhaps it was the cows getting such good grazing, or me being extra hungry, but whatever, it was especially delicious. We all mingled and talked and laughed and made friends and very thoroughly enjoyed ourselves.

After our fortifying lunch we went to buy a plant as a 'thank you' to Max and Giuseppe's parents and had a brief look round the small compact village. We found a beautiful, healthy specimen to all our satisfaction, then we went back and set off!

'Max's' Sentiero dei Fiori in October was a path surrounded by muted greens and fawns and browns. The sky above was a clear mid-blue, with puffy, drifting white clouds smoothly crossing it. They slowly thickened, increasing as we walked.

Max, our guide, left us in Giuseppe's capable hands, as he had a slight errand to run in the village, so the rest of us started. Giuseppe was keen to take us, knowing Max would catch us up easily, later.

The clearly defined mountain peaks in the distance looked like the contours of a gentle giant, lying down after a great feast and having a quiet doze. He seemed to be willing himself to take a much-needed nap.

There were no little multicoloured flowers that we could spot, but instead many strong tufts of hardy grass growing in clumps around the path. There were softly inclining slopes of dark-green bobbly conifers in the distance, a few scrubby trees close to hand, and what looked like having once been thistle-coloured flowers on tall willowy, wavy stems, gone to seed and shedding white, floaty fluff to the caring mountainside.

We marvelled at how the layers of soft greens and fawns and browns would recede mystically into the distance, with the clouds half covering them from view! We saw why Max had consistently urged us to hasten to visit these, 'his' mountains, which he loved so dearly.

Three-quarters of an hour on, we saw his sure lithe figure striding purposefully along towards us and we all sat down and became aware of breathing in deeply of that pure, invigorating air, while waiting for him to, at his own pace, cover the last uphill leg and join us.

We listened for him, and there was no noise at all. There was stillness and calm and peace. We were so comfortable after our warming meal, and, as Max arrived, we felt extremely happy.

The clouds drew in more as we returned, floating below us amongst the peaks and troughs, with small, spiky fronds of grass breaking up the dreamy mystery.

We said our goodbyes to Max and Giuseppe and family, piled dutifully into the car, took the special memories back to Conegliano, and said our farewells again. I'd gone home and had a shower, my heart warmed, and climbed readily into bed!

Chapter Two
February 1990

Eventually I tried coming downstairs from my bedroom very cautiously and gingerly. My chest was full of pain, a severe, unrelenting, mind-consuming soreness, and my legs were achy, weak and wobbly, but at least I was spending a few hours out of bed! Thus encouraged, I wondered if I'd soon be able to leave Ridlow, and get back home to Conegliano – and Dino, who so anxiously and kindly phoned me for a run down on my progress every week.

I sat down immediately I reached the lounge, glad to have walked a little, but half afraid I shouldn't have. I was in the chair next to my elderly, but sprightly grandmother, who was also feeling under the weather, with a virus of some sort sapping her strength. I was going to chat, but instead, as her head nodded slowly forward, I found my thoughts irresistibly returning to what had been, until so recently, my full and active life in Italy.

That memorable country walk from Cornuda to Asolo, with my good friends, in mid-November! The russets and burnt orange colours, golds and musky browns and gently sloping hillsides. The bare mountains behind them with snow on. Our peaceful picnic lunch, sitting, watching the still trees and candyfloss clouds spreading across the blue sky, and the warm companionship.

The skeletal trees had many fallen leaves and, like others waving daintily in the light breeze, they broke the firm line of the horizon, where the lower halves of the granite grey mountains sandwiched the white snow against the clear blue sky. The sun warmed our backs as we walked.

We'd reached the end of our outing, Asolo, at dusk, somewhat earlier than expected, then pottered interestedly round the busy antique market, looking up and admiring the darkened romantic castle, known as the Rocca, outlined above the trees at the top of the hill. That day it had seemed to me to be smiling benevolently down on the peaceful scene below.

Oh yes! That flame-like sunset edging out from behind the disparate clouds, with a promise of good weather for the morrow! Sitting down and taking it all in! Happily piling into cars and driving back home! And a good while later, in the evening, a visit to the uncrowded piano bar tucked discreetly away in Conegliano High Street with Dino. Sitting close and relaxed, exchanging our experiences of the day, unwinding and tapping our fingers to the music now and again, catching up. Leaving the bar as more people came in. The easy joy of seeing Dino again, of us both having our space to follow our own differing interests and never one condemn the other.

I suddenly came back to my home in Ridlow with a jolt. There was a loud knock at the front door. Some very good friends of the family had arrived. My parents welcomed them in, but I didn't know whether to go and greet them, as I couldn't possibly stay and chat to more than one person at a time, for more than a few minutes, and I felt embarrassed by the muddled words that might come out, as a result of my enfeebled mind. It was also very hard for me to stand up *and* talk at the same time.

Granny was wide awake now too, and she emphatically moved to the comfortable chairs in the dining room 'out of the way'... and I followed. It was incredibly stressful with so little energy saying "hello", then having to excuse yourself rapidly – my illness made me feel a need to be away from scrutiny and totally anonymous. I'd have braved the occasion if our good friends had not lived locally, but as it was we'd be sure to see each other again very soon. I just hoped that I might be more robust by then and able to share their company for a short while.

I sat still and softly whispered to Granny a little bit about my life in Italy. There was less vibration in my chest if I whispered, and so it was less painful than talking. I had to speak into Granny's ear though, as she was distinctly hard of hearing! I summoned up my last remaining strength before returning to bed and told her with pleasure about the cappuccino stops I'd sometimes made, with the little, round, meringue, almond cakes, which my clever parents and sister had 'discovered', when visiting. They'd noticed them on one of their holiday walks into the semi-arcaded Conegliano High Street. I recalled the shop was quite dark when you went inside, but that it didn't seem so by the time you ordered your drink. No extra was ever charged for sitting down at the tables, unlike a lot of coffee shops in Venice, for example, and there was a vast tempting array of melt-in-the-mouth little cakes to choose from! The sustaining cappuccinos there were large and good and frothy and had a nice lot of cocoa floating on the air bubbles. Sometimes I'd had a small espresso coffee, 'macchiato' with warmed frothy milk on top instead. That was it. Enough talking! I crawled up the stairs on my hands and knees and tumbled back into bed. I had to rest.

I was obliged to wait until the next day for more memories to float into my mind, because the effort I'd made made me weaker and obliterated everything but sheer pain all over. It was a relief to have my head clear a little, and see the coffee shop dance back into my thoughts, as I lay, trying to while the time away! I'd been able, after my family's fortuitous discovery, to take a couple of my English Viticulture students to have a drink there, towards the end of the course, when numbers had dwindled right down, through pressure of work, for our weekly conversation lessons. Instead of sitting talking inside the imposing meeting room of the Institute, we'd all walk down and have a good chat in English, with me jotting comments down, which we'd look at in detail while we enjoyed a cappuccino stop, finishing with a ten-minute walk and chat in English on the way back. One student in particular, Gianni, was very gifted, and he was especially disappointed I was planning to leave the Institute the following year and go to the more distant Venice University instead. I was just very sorry I couldn't fit it all in.

My thoughts moved on to the wonderful bread shop at the far end of my lovely road, right on the corner. Granny was an excellent, experienced, traditional cook and was thus extremely interested in good food! Next time I had a quiet chat with her, I'd see if she was interested in hearing about the *bread shop*! This particular shop always had row upon row of shiny or mottled loaves on display and the most delicious tempting smells wafting out as you stood still by the red traffic lights there, awaiting your eventual turn to cross the busy road.

I'd discovered wholesome walnut loaves in the bread shop and, sometimes, my good friend Richard, an English teacher too, and I would love to take some prepared buttered slices, or thick, unbuttered chunks for a tasty picnic along the stony, grassy banks of the River Piave - to eat with full-flavoured Grana or Provolone cheese, and Parma ham, and Italian apples.

Richard was tall and blond and very attractive! He had studied politics in London, and was also very good at French. Sometimes we inadvertently lapsed into French conversation - to practise! We were, in those days, after Umberto and I had separated, each other's trusted confidants, and freely listened and talked about life and love and our aspirations. I knew I was missing his company dreadfully. He was a really good friend.

I was still too weak to direct my thoughts, so I was thankful when the memories that came into my mind made me relatively cheerful, not sad, like when I thought about how severely I missed Dino and Richard. It was no good hankering to get back to Conegliano too soon. I had to let whatever illness I had run its course, and be more patient. At least I was now able to get up for an hour or so most days, and move downstairs for a change of scene.

There was nothing for it but to be thankful that my mind would wander back to the bread shop time and again! Andrea, my only sister, two years younger than me, had found she loved the place when she came to stay, not only because of the wafts of inviting crusty smells, but also as it was her 'landmark' when she was out and about walking in the town, reminding her of where to turn left to get back to my home.

Just a little further on from that corner was the health and fitness centre, where up until Christmas I'd been every week for my beloved evening jazz dance classes. It was just as well I did them, I'd always told myself, as there was also an especially tempting cake shop right opposite my flat!

My mother kindly brought me up my lunch, and asked me how I was feeling. I wished so desperately that there was some particular improvement that I could focus on, to cheer us all up, but there really wasn't. "Not too bad", I had to say, yet again, covering a multitude of aches and pains. I was trying to be positive and not dwell on them too much, hoping they'd take the hint and go away! My lungs were very sore, and the backs of my eyes were throbbing, so it was a relief after eating in the half-light of my bedroom (my 'head' couldn't stand the curtains more than a tiny bit drawn) to simply close my eyes and doze off once more.

Towards the end of February, my dear Italian neighbours, Maria and Sergio, came more often in to my mind. I'd first met them just over three years ago, when Umberto and I had moved in. I could see their lovely faces bobbing about in front of me at times! They must, I guessed, have been about ten years older than me – in their mid-forties. Maria was tall, slim and extremely attractive, wearing stylish, original, hand-made clothes. She came from Venice. Sergio, her husband, was also tall and striking and friendly, his hair greying, with a slight beard. I didn't normally like any 'fuzz on the chin', as my granny called it, but Sergio's beard suited his face perfectly. Both he and Maria were lively, and extremely kind and hospitable, looking after me like a sister. I loved them dearly, and as I lay there in Ridlow, although I had my kind mother and father and granny around me, and indeed my wonderful close friends Lizzie and Linda nearby, who generously drove over to see me for visits sometimes of no more than half an hour at a time, I still missed the sunshine and popping downstairs for my little heart-to-heart chats with my friendly Italian neighbours.

Sometimes Maria and Sergio entertained eight or more people to lunch or dinner, downstairs in their spacious taverna. Maria was a truly marvellous cook, preferring meat to fish dishes and doing wonderful pasta starters – as I'd found out, thanks to their generous invitations to me to join them and meet their friends.

The couple had suggested places to go to Umberto and me when we'd arrived in Conegliano, and we'd immediately taken them up on their wise counsel. Going to Eraclea by the sea, for example. There were sandy beaches, undulating dunes, maritime pine trees and the little town was quiet and clean. Several pizzerias stayed open throughout the year – just right for a snack lunch out of season – and we also liked it because it was less than an hour's drive away!

My friends Lizzie and Paul, and their little four year old, fair-haired son Jamie, had gone there with me for a sun and sea filled day when they came over on holiday. That lunchtime on the beach we'd become aware of two or three groups of mostly sun-tanned bodies 'gathering'. Lizzie, especially, had wondered aloud what was afoot. A savoury, briny, fishy smell was pervading the breeze, but nothing could be gleaned as to what was causing it! People then gradually began breaking away, holding plastic glasses filled with something red, and some small plates with food on. We swiftly went over to investigate and to our surprise found neat rows of sardines being char-grilled on a barbecue, and red or white local wine being poured out into the plastic glasses! It was all completely free, we found out – organised each year by the town hall, an exceptionally successful offering by the good people of Eraclea! We all duly queued up, being encouraged to do so by those already there, and gratefully received our three stripy fish and chunky white bread and red wine. It had been such a special day, and, as we tucked into our repast with alacrity, it seemed to me that the September sun was shining down approvingly on our experience! My memories of that occasion were warm-hearted and jolly, noisy and fun.

Eraclea, Eraclea... I'd once seen it from out at sea... the following year, from my good friend Davide's yacht – on which I'd kindly been invited for the day. I was so glad it was near enough to get to easily from Conegliano. I'd get back there and see it all again soon, I promised myself.

My thoughts remained with the Italian seasides that I had known up in the north of Italy. Of course! ...I would also from time to time journey to the chic Venice Lido beach... The reason for this was that I'd been fortunate enough to live in a sun-filled flat there for a happyish year whilst I was just getting to know Umberto, so it was quite nostalgic for me! It involved a fairly long trip from Conegliano, but had a completely absorbing and different atmosphere, so, when the mood struck, it was, I believed, well worth it. In the fullness of September, the renowned Leone D'Oro Cinema Prize was hotly contested there and the well-organised festival included amazingly individual and differing contributions from many interested nations. Participating actors and crew involved with the competing films would perhaps come and stay over at the grand and imposing Excelsior hotel, and there'd always be a buzzing, glamorous, slightly excited and anticipatory atmosphere on the exclusive sandy beach in front of it.

My travelling time from Conegliano to the Venice Lido was just over two hours! First I'd 'Venice walk', (fast and single-mindedly!), or drive my Uno to the elegant station. Then I'd relax once the train arrived, and take an hour's enjoyable ride. I'd sit by the window and watch Conegliano's undulating hills depart into the distance, as we chugged along, soon reaching the ribbon-like, meandering River Piave. My beloved flat was clearly visible as we went past! The fertile countryside would get considerably flatter as we pulled into

Treviso station after about half an hour, and I'd love gathering speed
after that and skimming on to industrial Mestre, knowing that from
that big, bustling, interchange station we'd have the joy of starting to
see the slightly algae-covered water and the uniquely beautiful
buildings that heralded the outskirts of Venice, in what seemed no
time at all. It was always my way to keep my eyes focused out of the
windows to see that first glimpse of Venice. Every time I found the
station building there a tiny bit smaller than I expected. For me it was
lively and welcoming. Then there was the fantastic sight walking out
and mingling with the atmosphere of this great city, the canal, the
people, the kiosks, the bridge and the domed church sunlit in front of
you.

I'd quickly hop on to a fast water bus or 'vaporetto', hoping I'd
see one coming as I arrived, for about forty joyous minutes, absorbing
what I could of Venice's beauty, and I'd happily arrive at the Lido!
Ten fast minutes' walk and I was finally on the sought-after beach!
Regularly *Death in Venice* came to mind, as I passed the somehow sad
Hotel des Bains.

One particular limpid summer's day, when I was living on the
Lido and Umberto and I were very close, my very kind and beautiful
friend Gabriella, and her charming pilot husband Michele, had invited
Umberto and I out for a memorable day on their splendid yacht.

I could picture now the golden glow of the warming summer sun
bathing everything in its light. The glint on Umberto's skin, as he
laughed, and how it seemed to take his cares away and lighten him, so
that I loved him even more – if that were humanly possible at that
time.

The fascinating dipping and raising of the clear, blue sea – ever in
motion and transforming itself into multifarious shapes urging, rather
than inviting, a brave, cooling, refreshing swim.

A courageous dip because of leaving that perfect, blissfully warm,
so comfortably relaxing and smoothly tactile wooden surface, that
made you think you might be a cat stretching contentedly.

It was so curious to me then to be bobbing gently a couple of
hundred metres offshore, and looking selectively, as though through a
wide-lensed microscope at the many still and moving figures on the
Excelsior beach. The sparkling water all around us had constantly
shone like a dimpled satin ribbon, a far-reaching flat one that flowed

out into the distance. There had been absolutely no sign of any fish, or tiny jellyfish either, just nearly tideless water.

There had been no fish to be seen either, when I'd been on my dear friend Davide's fantastic yacht rather later in the season, when the more defiant water already seemed greyer, and the feel of early autumn was just tingeing the crisper air – years on, when Umberto had gone.

At the Venice Lido with Gabriella and Michele, on that first generously offered day, Umberto had sometimes joked, easily and lightly laughed and warmly participated in the conversation. We could not have been made more welcome. Umberto told us stories of friends of his on yachts, and was full of exciting plans for the future, of finally finishing his civil engineering degree, and of finding exceptionally quickly a great job!

We'd plunged in, and dried off extremely quickly when sitting peacefully back on board! I'd been so extraordinarily happy, and taken in Umberto, almost in a detached and objective way – his strong, dark hair, and exquisitely formed face, with perfect white teeth that my grandmother so admired, his hairy chest and forearms, and slight, but at the same time, solidly robust frame. I'd known him a year then. I'd had no idea at that time of his impending claustrophobia, which was to break him away seven years later, and I could exactly recall the timeless joy on his face (and mine), as we were so deeply in love.

How utterly completely life can change…

Chapter Three
March 1990

At the beginning of March I was finally able to get up and go outside with my parents – just walking for a long fifteen minutes, which was, we all felt, a great and significant improvement. The necessary effort wore me out completely though, so at the same time it was rather depressing. I tried to tackle having to resign myself to taking much longer than I'd secretly hoped to get properly well. After the short walks, my dear mother, a young-looking, 'get up and go', sixty-three year old, with beautiful blue eyes and soft brown curly hair, and an inclusive and heart-warming smile, would ask me if I'd like to have a drink. How I'd have loved to have had something alcoholic to celebrate, but with my illness I didn't dare! Fizzy water or herbal tea was what I always asked for – mortified not to have the energy to go into the kitchen and find a glass or mug and pour it out or brew it for myself.

Time and again my thoughts drifted to Dino and other friends whom I missed more and more and I consciously pushed those memories away most of the time, unless I was feeling less fragile. I thought, somewhat nostalgically then, of 'Umberto's and my' bar in Conegliano – for we had moved up from the south of Italy together. We'd soon located it, although it was almost unnoticeable from the street! It was tucked away down our road, next to the busy health and dance centre. The owner, I recalled, prided himself on the wide variety of different beer he kept available, and offered exquisitely filled warm toasted sandwiches in lovely crispy bread – the melted cheese, with a good helping of prosciutto crudo and a dash of mustard turned out to be our favourite. There'd been, when we'd first discovered this our local, long, spaced-off, sturdy wooden tables, with polished wooden benches rather than chairs either side. I think the place, novel for Italy, reminded Umberto of Germany or England, and that was one of the main reasons he liked it so much.

Mostly, we'd noticed, young groups of people seemed to go there and at every table you could see they were having something tasty to eat, as well as Coke to drink. Perhaps the hardened beer lovers came in later, when we'd gone!

We went off the trusty bar somewhat when they overly smartened it up, putting in brighter lights, exchanging benches for chairs, and opening up the less inviting back, which was still rather dark and gloomy to our minds, although it made the eating area bigger. The only good thing we could see about the improvements was that there were now on offer some delicious spaghetti dishes as well as the sandwiches, at a very competitive price.

Our local bar had had a boxed-off pay phone, which had been extremely useful when Umberto and I first moved in, both for calls to England and Italy, and that was surprisingly got rid of during the refurbishment – probably, we reckoned, because we'd used it too much and had had to interrupt long, deep and flavoursome conversations at the bar in order to pay!

It was homely though, that bar, and really down-to-earth when we first knew it, with a solid, comforting and dependable feel! It was not other-worldly at all, not like the enchanting place that had been so long our favourite in Venice, as we were getting to know each other, Ai Specchi. That bar was smaller and more intimate, and the four walls were completely covered in beautiful old mirrors, of varied curved and harmonious shapes and sizes. It gave the room a mystical atmosphere on long, dark evenings! Wherever you sat, you could not fail to take the mirrors and collage of reflections in. They caught the light, which flickered and changed in hue as customers went in and out.

There was a small wooden shelf in Ai Specchi, high at the top of the wall, all the way round the room, with finished and half-consumed bottles of bourbon and whiskey on. Apparently some of the richer regular customers would buy their own bottles and keep them separately up there for the next time.

In that magical phase of our lives, Umberto and I had gone now and again to Ai Specchi, and always ordered, for some reason, despite our impoverished state, a bourbon and ginger ale! Everywhere else we drank wine or beer or water. We'd watch closely, fascinated, as the extremely able barman would lovingly prepare our long drinks in tall glasses, with plenty of ice, and a fresh sprig of mint, with a tremendous flourish! Even if you were not looking directly at him, you could follow his deft expertise in the mirrors!

The barman at Ai Specchi often got called upon by other thirsty customers to prepare exotic cocktails, and the stainless steel shaker would be used to much effect, but our particular long drinks would be swiftly stirred with a brightly coloured red or orange plastic rod, with a small, moulded animal on the top, and these would be left in the glasses for us to continue rattling the ice as we sipped our special drinks! In harmony, Umberto and I would absorbedly talk at length and make what we believed to be wholesome, tangible plans for the future – that wasn't to be.

Eight years of compromises and application... all gone. Perhaps, I tried to reassure myself positively now, when I got well, my future was to be spent happily with Dino? I knew that I really hoped so, because both he and I were getting over our failed marriages, and we enjoyed each other's company so much. I might have little more trouble getting over my illness once the warmer weather arrived, and get back to Conegliano quickly, and see him soon! Maybe Umberto leaving because his claustrophobia made him feel he couldn't cope with married life had all been for the best?

My day-dreaming, restless mind travelled purposefully back to the piano bar, tucked away in the centre of Conegliano, which I'd never even noticed until I met Dino. How did that compare? Well, it was spacious, entertaining with its variety of live music, and it was elegant! Just like Dino! You sank thankfully into the soft, low seats, comfortably sensing yourself blend in to the background, as the soft lighting was romantic, and merged all the hard outlines together, or, rarely, you perched rather self-consciously on high bar stools, in the bright light around the piano!

That was one thing, I remembered – soft seats in the Conegliano piano bar *were* available and, at Ai Specchi, glamorous and intriguing though the wrought-iron chair backs had been, they and the seats were hard to start with, and they became harder throughout the evening!

I smiled ruefully to myself as I suddenly thought of our very *own* bar, Umberto's and mine – at home! To the right as you entered our square lounge in our flat in Conegliano had been the very first, caringly chosen piece of furniture that we'd rashly gone out and bought in Caserta when we got married! We'd sincerely gone out to choose a useful washing machine, with my Granny's wedding present money – and we'd both unexpectedly fallen in love with our large, attractive, wooden, weathered-looking old bar! It had a tall, shelved, dresser-like back and a shiny, polished, serving surface, hiding more useful storage space beneath. The front had soft orange leather trimmings, which sunnily drew your gaze.

Umberto and I had talked ourselves into buying that wooden bar, thinking it could stand in our lounge as a variation on a more traditional sideboard! As it turned out, that was fortunately a successful move, as it was well used when any friends dropped in, and it could hold a marvellous amount of books out of sight, as well as displaying a colourful, cheering and decorative array of drinks and glasses!

The chestnut was rounded and threw out feelings of well-being. Just at the top of the bar, on the back, there sparkled a small mosaic of mirrors, which caught the light in the evenings, and twinkled into the whole room, reminding us of Ai Specchi. On the slightly dipping shelves, wine and spirits, (grappa from Umberto's family and brandy from mine amongst them), would make shadows in the mirrors' reflected light.

The first time I'd come home to England for a summer holiday, after purchasing the bar, I'd eventually found the necessary hour or so to make long, narrow, pale-blue towelling shelf liners, and the glasses, many being lovely wedding presents, now lay on them. I liked our long drink glasses best – with a painted orange stork at the bottom, standing close to a red and orange and yellow setting sun! I also had a soft spot for the milky white cocktail glasses I'd found as a bargain hunter in Italy! These became clear as if by magic when any liquid was placed in them, but looked frosted, as though with sugar, around the dry tops!

When friends came round, most preferred to settle for wine, although I'd concocted some wonderful iridescent blue cocktails with curaçao in my time! I'd also done red or pink ones with Campari when my friend Jill, a good and trusted teacher friend from New Zealand dropped in, as Campari was her favourite. I could picture the lounge in Conegliano with us all sitting there. The seating arrangement was varied! Some people would perch apparently precariously on the two orange, leather-covered stools by the front of the wooden bar, others might sink cautiously but comfortably into our bumper peachy and blue, sandy and sea-coloured rough silk cushions on the floor, and the luckiest would head for the one and only sofa!

Maria and Sergio would come and join Umberto and me quite often when we first moved in. They said over a welcoming get-together several times that they really must take us for an afternoon 'giro' – an outing to see some picturesque places in and around Sergio's birthplace of Conegliano. Then, after a busy couple of months, they found time to take us on the wonderful promised excursion. Curiously their car was identical to ours; an Opal Kadett, silver, with a blue stripe along the side, so sitting in it felt perfectly natural!

We were taken for a meandering drive through the sunny, hazy hills, many covered in spectacular vineyards – beautifully sunlit and shaded, and restfully calm and peaceful.

We stopped first at Conegliano's medieval castle for a much-appreciated glass of chilled sparkling prosecco wine, sitting on the outside terrace, taking in the grey stone walls and the vast expanse of trees and grass and red-brown roof-tops below. Then, without haste, we were taken to the small, idyllic watermill at Refrontolo, where the wheel slowly turned, and you felt as though you were in an oil painting, and could picture yourself skipping across the stones to the other side of the trickling stream!

Just up the steeply sloping hill and round the next corner, we'd gone to the shady, vine-covered, dappled, wooden tables and benches of a favourite restaurant of Maria and Sergio's, which was renowned amongst local people, and served a delicious 'coffee special'. Local grappa, espresso coffee and a secret ingredient were combined into a warm glassful of power and delight – we'd had *two*! The steep slope up to the restaurant looked much like a private entrance, so the popular place was effectively hidden away from those who did not know!

We'd all had such a great time travelling round and finishing up at Castel Brandolini, where in the stillness of its tree-filled courtyard, whilst looking down at the tops of the magnificent evergreens on the hillside below, we'd understood why many people, young and old, came there for a spiritual retreat.

Back came my mind to Ridlow, and I concentrated on where I was while we had lunch! Afterwards I had a swift, passing thought about trying to go for a very short walk with my father, to get some fresh air, and be briefly out of the house. How I would have dearly loved to! But I was so up and down, and this was one of the days I really wasn't up to it. Not even for five minutes. My father went for his daily walks as regularly as clockwork! He was a tall, distinguished, handsome man in his sixty-fifth year, but nobody would ever have guessed it! To my mind he looked at least fifteen years younger. More than one of my friends had said he strongly reminded them of a striking Vincent Price in his early years!

Our beautiful, sweet-natured golden retriever, Rusty, would go walking with my father. She was named by Granny after her rippling, wavy, shining coat, and she'd adore her regular forty minute outing straight after lunch! Admittedly she'd go more willingly some days than others, but once she got going, we could rely on her to really enjoy herself, picking up her pace, and finding large stones to carry!

Sadly there was nothing for it. I went exhaustedly into the warm, comfortable dining room, and joined my grandmother who was totally absorbed doing some lovely, colourful, patterned tapestry, having recovered from her virus, and plonked down in an armchair for ten minutes, before returning to bed. Granny was eighty-six, and had fine, grey hair permed into a fetching round shape that suited her face. We were naughty sometimes, and called her 'Sheepy sheep'! She had a good sense of humour, and we often had a laugh, especially if she'd made a funny mistake in conversation! Being so hard of hearing, she quite often got hold of the wrong end of the stick. "Would you like a cup of tea?", for example, could even be interpreted as "Do you really want a wee?" Or "Rusty's just there – be careful", as "Crusty bread's cheap and cheerful"!

Granny was very generous, and I remembered her warm hospitality right back from when she still lived in her tidy little flat in Ipswich, before moving into my parents' in Ridlow. She had been known to give us occasional aperitifs of gin and mixed Martini cocktails (with a cherry in) that made us all but stand on our heads! I was always reminded of flowers, too, when I thought of Granny, as in her own home she would lovingly pick fresh roses or other beautiful blooms from the garden to grace her living-room mantelpiece in small, dainty, silver vases!

After ten minutes I had to go. It was depressing feeling ten times worse than the day before. As very often I had to crawl upstairs on my hands and knees again, and, though lonely in my room, take refuge there, for I had no more energy within me to be able to communicate further with anyone at all. Thoughts were suspended too, as a searing pain tore at the left side of my head.

Relief next morning to see Maria and Sergio's kind faces swim faintly into my muzzy mind and find the headache only half as bad. I quietly remembered going with them from Conegliano to the beautiful, (and popular for weddings), lightly imposing abbey at Follina! I had, in England, a photo they'd taken of me standing happily by the small columns, dressed for summer in a favourite pink and red and green flowery blouse. It perfectly matched the geraniums in the long window boxes that ran gaily and uniformly along the waist-high wall of the cloisters!

There'd been, I recalled, at the time of that our first visit, a traditional wedding going on there, and so we'd only peeked in to the abbey, and then pottered round the tranquil cloisters, admiring the covered well in the centre. I'd been very grateful to be shown the beauty of Follina, because, amongst other things, when Linda and Lizzie and her family had come over from Cambridge on holiday, we'd immediately been able to go there and enjoy its absorbing splendour!

I had, upstairs, a photo of Linda and Eric and me, standing together at the picturesque watermill at Refrontolo. Thanks to Maria and Sergio's wonderful guided tour, showing me where these places were, I'd been able to take them there, and my family all round as well! I felt distinctly queasy, but sipped at the lemon water by my bed, and willed myself to dig out that picture – and it brought back the happy memories vividly!

Linda, bonny, fair-skinned, blonde and blessed with a wonderful bubbly personality, was an English language teacher, like me, and Eric had been one of our gifted foreign students in Cambridge on a short summer course. Eric was Belgian, and had come to northern Italy on holiday with all his family, near Conegliano. Linda had spontaneously suggested we take him out for an "unforgettable day", not leave him on the beach for a whole week! So we had hoped to do! We'd had a great, firmly established rapport and much fun from the moment we met up. Linda was extremely outgoing, forthright, and such good company, a real lover of the whole of Italy, and so was Eric!

We'd all gone to Refrontolo first, and so much enjoyed the quiet, secluded atmosphere. Linda had suggested we go there for a change from the meandering River Piave for a picnic! The mill wheel turned slowly behind the three of us and a powerful car had noisily arrived. We'd asked if that elderly driver would take our photo – and here it was, in my hand!

We'd lingered awhile and talked and reminisced, and then the time drew on, and we knew we soon must part, perhaps never to meet up again. There'd been nothing for it – we'd all just *had* to go up the hill, round the corner, for a warming, welcoming, albeit wintry grappa 'coffee special', to wish each other happiness in the future, before visiting the sunlit abbey at Follina, which rounded off our lovely day!

Chapter Four

April 1990

I was able to go for a slightly longer walk of twenty minutes at the beginning of April, and even joined my family for a very short trip to town, walking one day for ten minutes around Boots – which was heavenly after so much time at home, despite my wobbly, aching legs! I was hopeful I could really enjoy my granny's birthday on April 7th. She would be eighty-seven! I wasn't too bad on the 6th, then, hey presto, my temperature went up again and I felt full of flu once more when I woke up on the 7th. How frustrating! I wasn't going to be beaten though, and I rested quietly all the morning and thankfully felt much better by twelve o'clock.

Every day was a challenge, but this was a particular one. Granny had always had an exceptionally sweet tooth, and loved chocolates, but now surprised us all, having gone off them altogether! So I'd asked my younger sister if she'd kindly get me a navy neck scarf to go with Granny's suit and some light perfume for me to give her. Some fairly distant relations were coming over for a cold buffet lunch to mark the occasion. I went downstairs and joined everyone as they arrived, and tried to chat despite my aching trachea and sore lungs. I managed for an hour, and willed myself to stay for longer, but I found I still hadn't the energy to concentrate on eating and making polite conversation at the same time. I had no alternative but to reluctantly retire to my room, as the rasping pain in my chest was aggravated beyond belief when I spoke, and my temperature had gone up again.

It was no good. I seemed doomed to be unable to participate much in anything for the time being. I was always having to go and rest, and, as a matter of course, my anxious brain still returned me urgently, and apparently of necessity, to Conegliano, which I had had to leave so unprepared, as soon as I lay down quietly on my own.

Who would have thought that coming home for the Christmas holiday would have led to *this*?

I couldn't help but keep on thinking of Dino and my friends, but now I was really frightened that I might take a long time to get well, because of making so little progress, and it upset me even more. My mind kept returning to Italy anyway, so I pushed away the most painful memories, and concentrated on lighter reminiscences.

I was able to think nostalgically of Linda and Eric once more on the day we'd shared together, and of the good laughs we'd had even when taking Eric slowly back to rejoin his more retiring family in popular Jesolo! We'd all gingerly and deftly picked a 'stop start' way through the bunched lines of brown and not so brown bodies lying and sitting relaxed on the barely visible, sandy beach! We'd been sincerely surprised at quite how many happy, holidaying people there still were, even though the lowering and fading afternoon sun was drawing on. The rippling sea had been fully dotted with adept and cautious swimmers, and seemingly light-hearted, fun-loving people in red and chrome paddle boats, barely moving, rather bobbing chirpily about over the inviting, gentle waves. Linda had looked in horror, as she wasn't, in her own self-aware words, a "beach person" anyway, and so we'd reluctantly said our goodbyes and then driven in my green Fiat Uno back to my flat, for a restorative and welcome plate of appetisingly, thinly sliced Parma ham, and crunchy, tasty, mixed salad, with plenty of local radicchio and small, peppery leaves of rocket!

Another very good day with Linda also came back to me, mercifully distracting, as I tried, with practised achievement, if not ease, to wholly concentrate on something other than the sore, aching, fevered pain of my limbs and raging trachea! ...The extra effort I'd made was taking its toll again. Ah yes, it had been a Friday – market day in Conegliano, and we'd happily walked round the many varied, bargain-filled stalls, making the occasional purchase, like a multicoloured, abstract, predominantly blue skirt for Linda, and two portions of plump, grey, meaty prawns, to fry up as a special treat, with a more heavily handed addition of tasty garlic than I would have put in for myself alone!

Linda and I had successfully met up with Umberto that Friday. Although Umberto and I had been sadly separated for a year, and didn't see much of each other, he thankfully was still very fond of dear Linda, and she of him, so the three of us were happy to all get together. Umberto, that evening, had generously and kindly taken us to an exclusive fish restaurant out in the Veneto countryside, called Feltrin – where the main speciality, amongst a wide selection of extremely good food, was freshwater crayfish. I'd heard excellent tales of the distinctive place before, and was certainly very curious to try it!

Linda and I had spent an enjoyable, 'pottering' afternoon beforehand, sightseeing in elegant and accessible Treviso, both dressed unremarkably casually, and even, if we were honest, a shade crumpledly – rather more than usual! Umberto had soon met us, particularly cheerfully, rather smarter and more elegant in his well-chosen, tasteful clothes, and he'd sprung the appealing and tempting idea of the special fish meal out on us late, so we didn't have time to go back to our base in Conegliano and change!

So we'd thought for half a second, and said, "Yes" to his kind invitation, though we didn't feel we were at all dressed for the occasion! Our first thought when we'd arrived at the restaurant had been to talk long and happily in English to start with, hoping we could get away with looking semi-scruffs, because we were foreign! Umberto was exceedingly good and didn't look embarrassed or ill at ease – despite the strong emphasis he put on being correctly dressed for every occasion, and we all soon forgot our keenly felt self-consciousness when the delicious food arrived!

The parchment menu we were handed was written in Pompeiian red ink, in local dialect, and it extremely comprehensively explained the best way of approaching and eating "mouth-watering crayfish"! The attentive, black-jacketed waiter was thrilled to hand us a menu in English too!

When Linda and I looked at the English translation, we were unable to suppress our amusement completely. We had to try our best to satisfactorily explain our merry mirth to our kind, bemused host, Umberto! Our best, because it was almost impossibly hard for us to get across in my everyday Italian, for example, that "tear off its paws" just wouldn't be likely to be written in an English fish restaurant menu! The word order was distinctly and joyfully odd, the welcome guide to eating saying that intrepid diners should "lay aside customary formalities and set purposefully aside both fork and knife". Then the poor crayfishes' "paws", as we read delightedly on, certainly tickled our sense of humour and drew most of our attention! We all eventually gleaned, Umberto as well, that after we'd successfully torn off the "limp, hanging paws", it was necessary to squash the great ones with teeth in order that we could taste the inside meat!

The "tasty morsel's" shell became the presumed "crust", and we were to put a nail of ours at the end of this crust, and where the tail had its origins, *raise* it to reach the golden morsel! Having got there, we were instructed: "Give it up"!

We had such a warm, close, unexpectedly good time, filled with shared laughter and delight, and it was a deeply fitting way for lovely Linda and kind-hearted Umberto to say goodbye to each other, as, fate decreeing, they never saw a glimpse of each other again.

We'd driven home to Conegliano, Linda and I, slowly and carefully, each the proud owners of an oatmeal-coloured pottery plate with 'Feltrin' and a crayfish drawn on in brown paint, by hand.

The severe pain in my chest was thankfully easing and I really felt a lot more relaxed and sociable and comfortable. But I still stayed tucked right away in my peaceful, quiet forest glade, until our welcome guests had gone, as I unfortunately knew from experience that I'd immediately feel a very great deal worse again if I threw caution to the winds and went straight back down, because it would strain my weakest spots talking and concentrating too hard. I'd always appreciated company, so I was sincerely sorry to have to stay lying down resting, alone in my bedroom, removed from the action.

Rusty, interrupting my thoughts, gentle and beloved of all the family, came padding cautiously round the door to see and cheer me for a short while. Her beautiful silky soft coat ranged from a darker rust colour on her head and back, to a lighter, feathery beige underneath, and around her tail. She lay down contentedly beside me, stretching out her lean front paws, panting with her pink, curled tongue poking out a little, then, after about ten minutes, she wagged her tail slowly a couple of times, and got up deliberately on to all fours again, wending her way purposefully right across the room, a tiny bit side-tracked to the left by the inviting waste-paper basket, but soon passing through the green ajar door, and softly back downstairs!

Once more I was alone, and left to my imaginary world of the past to liven up the present. And, wondering where to cast my mind, I suddenly alighted upon the beautiful city of Florence. Yes... of course! I'd been there on a memorable, action-packed day trip from Conegliano with Jill, and for two equally action-packed and exciting days with my parents and sister! I'd also keenly studied spoken Italian there for four months in my younger student days. I'd been wholly entranced by the powerful, engaging art and the harmonious architecture each and every fortuitous time I was there.

The wonder of fireflies came vividly back to me, appearing and disappearing, dancing gaily and merrily, as if totally carefree, all around me as I walked, entranced, down to the splendour of Florence from the spacious Piazzale Michelangelo, and I felt how it had almost seemed to me I'd been magically transported for half an hour to fairyland! I'd heard the noisy grating of crickets as I passed by, which added to the wonderful atmosphere.

And one fine summer day I'd been calmly walking down from the Fortezza da Basso at about half past five, after studying for the afternoon quietly up there, in the cool, breezy grounds, and an ungainly, burly man had approached me on a smallish, noisy motorbike! He'd indicated forcefully that he wanted me to get on the back of it, and when I had vehemently shaken my head and backed off, he'd become aggressive, insistent, grabbing hold of my right forearm hard and forcing me completely off the road and into the bushes along the side.

That was undoubtedly the very first time I had been terrifically scared of something other than painful illness, and I was so unutterably relieved when, merely seconds later, a young Florentine girl who was also walking calmly down the sloping road, with her large, beautiful and protective Alsatian, had swiftly seen my very real predicament and unhesitatingly come running to my aid. The cowardly man had taken one good look and immediately revved up his motorbike, fumbled to point it down the hill, and fled. And so Ilarea, for that was her name, and I were to be very close for my last couple of studying days in Florence, before I returned to England.

When, years after that regrettable incident, I'd been to Florence in the June of '87, from Conegliano, with my holidaying parents and Andrea, I'd been glad not to be going there on my own again. It was also great, I thought, to have transport! We went by car.

The four of us arrived in Florence in good time after a morning's drive, to find each of the narrow roads we travelled down hopefully jam-packed along both pavements with parked cars, and the volume of

Florentine traffic more daunting and nerve-racking than I remembered! We already had the name and address of the small pension with *a garage*, where we were booked in advance to stay the night – the only trouble was reaching it. We spent what seemed like *hours* trying desperately to follow the one-way systems around to 'our' road. We were always nearby, but it was well nigh impossible at most stages to turn the car round, and the one-way streets weren't indicated on our map!

Miraculously, we did eventually arrive, and we thankfully left the car in the pension garage, from then on all going out sightseeing on foot! Even my dear mother braved her sometimes aching leg and abandoned four wheels! My father, lieutenant during the Second World War in the 17/21st Lancers regiment, known as the 'Death or Glory Boys', had been posted for a few weeks just south of the city of Florence, and it brought him back many varied, happy, and nostalgic memories.

Walking round the sights, we'd graduated to the lovely Ponte Vecchio, which spanned the River Arno, that was low with slow-moving water, and there my father bought my mother a very carefully chosen gold and silver eternity ring, with small sparkling diamonds on, from one of the several gold jewellery shops picturesquely lining the crowded bridge! She left her gold wedding ring to be slightly enlarged too, as it was squashing her ring finger, and, after a much-anticipated and heart-warming visit to the splendid church of Santa Croce, the beautiful paintings in the Uffizi gallery and the classical, stately statues and steps of the Boboli gardens, we all returned, sprightly in our steps, to the bustling Ponte Vecchio, and my mother picked the ring up, wondering how it would be… and it was perfect!

Chapter Five
May 1990

Lying still, wide awake at five thirty in the morning, I straight away realised I was feeling – in every way – much better than I had done so far, ever since my distressing illness had started. A good friend of my grandmother's was due to be coming for a roast beef lunch, and I calmly resolved to, as always, try and join in with everyone as much as possible! I had spent fifteen absorbing, but tiring minutes the previous evening sorting out my precious, heavy albums of photos, some of the family and some of Italy, to show Milli if she liked, and I was sincerely hoping I'd get that far and wouldn't need to return to my room, albeit so much a haven, or need to rest while she was here.

The green, dappled light was dancing rhythmically on the pale green cupboard door, as the first spring leaves gently blocked the bright early morning sun's promisingly powerful rays. And glancing in all directions around the room, my eyes, darting, I felt, in time with the bobbing leaves, were drawn to a pair of beautiful gold clasped earrings, which I'd only worn recently – clear, enamel-coated, miniature Aspen leaves, from Aspen in Colorado, picked at just the right stage in the fall to give a mellow, golden glow – my parents had kindly given me them one year, after a wonderful holiday they'd had there, along with my sister Andrea. I had a gold dragon too, lying on the wooden chest, depicted on enamelled white and turquoise stone, a compact and also 'natural' gift, unusual and attractive, attached to a light, auburn leather thong. It was from Andrea, also from Aspen, a place she loved so dearly and so well. Looking at those gifts, and being reminded of the beauty of Colorado, which I had heard so much about, I looked forward to the possibility of maybe one day seeing the place for myself. *If I could get completely better!* My eyes next alighted on a neat silver brooch, pink and purple hues swirled in the silver, a timeless Mexican butterfly, open winged and ready to flit away, from Linda. Linda and I would buy each other a small souvenir gift from our holidays, and we had enjoyed so many together!

In Orvieto, in Italy, near the spectacular Duomo, with its breathtaking multicoloured mosaics of the Creation and biblical prophesies on the front façade, and the rich, powerful Signorelli frescoes of the Apocalypse inside, Linda and I, when wandering round the busy streets, one holiday together, after Umberto and I had separated, the early evening sun lowering and filling the town with a promising orangey-red light, had both spotted a large earthenware container for flour, and Linda had bought it for me as a 'thank you' for us travelling round in my car! It was about ten inches high and eight inches wide, off-white, with the Italian word 'Farina' written in clear, flowing letters on the front, in Mediterranean blue.

For many years at the back of my mind, I'd been dreaming of just such a flour holder! It reminded me of the old-fashioned spacious walk-in English pantries and my granny's delicious home baking! I'd taken it proudly back to my smallish flat in Conegliano, and stood it carefully, where I'd already pictured it, near the south-facing kitchen window, so it easily caught the daylight and generally the admiring attention of the many friends who might pop round the wooden door to see what was cooking! The Orvieto flour container stood on the smooth, white, marble worktop, contrasting with the dark oak cupboards, an ever-ready and handy reminder for *me* to do some baking. Luckily, in case of mishaps, there was the excellent cake shop over the road from my flat to fall back on!

Every year in Italy at Christmas I attempted to make my classes of English students individual mince pies. However these turned out, they were cooked with love, in relays! And so, amazingly, the 'comfortable' flour would get used up!

In Orvieto, on our travels, I'd happily bought Linda a lovely octagonal tin for keeping her various tea bags in! She'd chosen it in preference to earthenware. She wanted something light and practical, she told me, and after we'd looked everywhere we could think of, we'd eventually found the pretty tin that was predominantly orange and green and blue, cut up fruit appetisingly depicted on its sides and lid – perfect, Linda thought, for herbal fruit teas!

I had seen neither similar tins, nor earthenware containers in Conegliano's excellent and well-stocked shops, whilst occasionally ambling round, although in nearby central Treviso I'd soon spied some similar cream earthenware in a shop window. I didn't honestly like it as much as the one which Linda had generously bought me – and in Treviso it was more expensive!

Another reason I'd been so pleased to receive that blue and off-white flour container, was that I'd been thinking for a while I'd like to have more blue in my kitchen! I'd been interested when Linda and I had visited my good friend Sarah at her picturesque house in the medieval hilltop town of Stroncone, in Umbria – for she had a completely blue and white kitchen, in varying shades, that looked fresh, and alive, and very engaging!

Sarah was always so hospitable and kind, and we'd enthusiastically taken up her invitation to stay a couple of August days with her and her charming family, before returning to Conegliano. I could close my eyes tightly now, in Ridlow, and clearly see us all, feeling so at home, sitting in that summery blue and white kitchen, with a beautiful view of the valley falling away below – and in the kitchen, the wooden table, covered abundantly in small pine nuts in their light brown shells, which we were all busily cracking, ready to make without a doubt the most delicious fresh pesto sauce I had ever eaten! The smooth, elongated, oval, white nuts seemed to make an incredibly minuscule amount of food to eat without their protective shells on for what seemed like hours, so more and more were systematically cracked, and finally we had worked up an enormous appetite, and looked benignly upon a substantial pile of pine kernels in the round dish, ready to mix and crush with the perfumed basil, the tasty Pecorino cheese, the plump juicy garlic and the emerald green virgin olive oil!

Stroncone, the picturesque place where Sarah lived for a couple of months every summer, was truly a joy to visit! It couldn't be expanded upon with modern concrete or brick buildings, as it was walled, and there was no more room for expansion to go. We happened to be there for the marvellous celebration of the town's renowned Beato Angelico, who was reverently taken in his glass coffin, his small, peaceful body visible to us all, through the narrow streets, and I had an abiding sense of his journey now, as I thought back to it. A group of ladies had lined up as darkness descended, and leant right over one of the waist-high walls in front of us, to better see the religious procession making its way along the straight road from the church below, so, looking for a good vantage point, we had had a view first of a row of white illuminated legs and rounded behinds! Sarah had urged me to snap the shot quickly and preserve it for posterity!

As we'd stood waiting for and watching the procession, from the light of the street lamps behind, we'd noticed the attractive stone arches and medieval walls of Stroncone being that beautiful weathered combination of pale greys and browns and yellows, blending into one layered, mottled whole – a wise whole, I believed, having withstood so much of life!

Linda and I had really felt refreshed when we returned to Conegliano, Veneto shortly afterwards. We took our photos along to my local photographic shop straight away, barely able to contain our curiosity as to how they'd turn out, and got them developed! I was so glad I had them to dip into now!

The photographs jogged my memory about some very lovely places in the north of Italy that had been visited by Linda and me a year later too! Bassano del Grappa came to mind, at the foot of the impressive Monte Grappa, with its green river, and the ancient red-roofed houses. Linda, and my close friends Massimo, Carlo and Isobella, along with my jazz dance teacher Marta, and her two friends Jacopo and Enrico, had gone there for the day. I looked at us all in a group, standing on the old wooden bridge; the Ponte degli Alpini, and leaning against the balustrades, with the river and mountains in the background, while we gaily took each other's photos! We'd all linked arms and smiled, looking forward, I remembered, to sampling a small drop of one of the enormous variety of grappas on offer at the attractive bar next door!

Walking around Bassano, we'd earlier come across a poor young pigeon, fluffy and frightened, which had apparently fallen off a window ledge from the second floor, and although seeming quite big, it didn't seem able to fly and get out of the way of the people and, worse still, the traffic. Carlo had carefully picked it up, and thrown it upwards towards the empty window ledge it had come from, three or four times, hoping it would settle back safely, but it didn't. In the end we'd put it away from the traffic and passing people, on the inner side of the pavement on some grass, and reluctantly left it, hoping that when not so much the centre of attention, later in the day, it would be able to find somewhere better still.

That fluffy young bird had been so vulnerable and we'd been reluctant to leave it. In some way, it reminded me of another outing of nine of us in September '87, two and a half years ago. My kind neighbours Maria and Sergio had organised a fantastic and much-looked forward to walk, up in the green, chestnut-covered hills to the no longer inhabited castle of Mel, perched on a woody hilltop! There wasn't a cloud in the bright blue sky that day, either, and I recalled we'd set off from sunny Conegliano on Sunday morning at nine o'clock, relaxed, and fit, and full of expectation!

We'd travelled through the nearby Passo San Boldo, which was rough and bumpy for the cars, and soon to be closed for repair, as it turned out, and stopped eventually at an unexpected, isolated, homely looking *osteria*, called Pan e Pit, where fresh chicken and polenta (the typical northern Italian dish of semolina-like dough cooked with cornmeal flour), was swiftly ordered for our expected return at about four thirty in the afternoon; a late lunch!

Sergio and one of his good friends had slipped away and gone to help choose the chicken we would be eating, while it ran happily with the others around the large, earthen yard. For some reason that chicken was linked in my mind with the little pigeon in Bassano!

We'd had a lively and entertaining walk, much interesting conversation, and we'd so enjoyed getting out into the wonderful countryside – we'd stopped and paddled a while in a small, clear, shallow, fast-moving stream, and I had felt very lucky to be seeing these beautiful, peaceful, hidden-away places I would never have got to on my own! The chestnuts stained our fingers when we stopped and prized some open, and, as we made our way back to the Pan e Pit, like horses whose paces quicken as they near home, we found ourselves striding out more, and our appetites growing.

That chicken, gently and tastily casseroled on an open log fire, along with the constantly stirred straw-coloured polenta, in its large, metal container, all perfumed with the smoke from the burning wood, was utterly delicious. We appreciated every mouthful. I loved the togetherness round the table, sharing the sumptuous meal, but at the same time it made me vow inwardly to myself that I would try and eat less meat in future. Just as, strangely enough, the episode with the pigeon had done.

Chapter Six
June 1990

The beginning of June, and again I spent the morning stuck in bed upstairs, with aches and pains and a very bad migraine-like headache, white and coloured lights zigzagging backwards and forwards crazily in front of my eyes. I couldn't believe I was *still* here in England, housebound!

Just before lunch my kind parents drove me to nearby Newmarket, for a first hastily arranged, expert acupuncture treatment. Six months of this illness, and the medical doctors had only been able to do a few tests and offer nothing to help me at all. I barely winced when the fine, glistening steel needles went swiftly, for just a moment, into both my temples, my lower tummy and feet – and my poor head felt the pain lift slightly, and my limbs ached less. It had been an effort getting there, but with the significant relief of my symptoms it was worth it!

Later in the day, in the sunny afternoon, I was to find I had enough energy to enable me to leave my sad, quiet, dark room, and sit out in the garden for a change. Sitting, rather than lying flat didn't wear me out after an hour or so as it usually did, and I was able to bear noise slightly better. I even watched some ballet on the television, and it reminded me of when I'd been able to dance.

For the first time I was able to cast my mind back to those days – a hitherto impossible task, as no longer being able to walk about freely had wounded my heart to the core. I must, I thought, be healing a bit inside too, to be able to face such memories better! Dino, on one of his rare 'free' weekends, and some other good friends had joined me only a year ago to watch Marta's spectacular end of term dance show! A year before that, in June of '88, I'd been dancing in it myself! I'd longed to sit in the audience and spectate, rather than fight my pre-show nerves, and in June of '89 I was so much busier, I had what I hoped was a valid excuse that I hadn't really got the necessary time to rehearse, (although I'd practised the routines in classes) – and so, in June of '89 I'd been able to join my friends in the auditorium!

I wished I could bring those times back! Magic away my daily reality! Dino had sat quietly beside me, tall and lithe, with his mid-length, slightly wavy, light brown hair framing his strikingly slim and beautiful face. He was like a fashion model! He always dressed with great care and attention, achieving a sporty, classic look, and turned many heads when he walked by. I had been going out with him for nine months then and from our cautious beginnings, we'd become much more relaxed and easy and secure in our relationship.

Jill had sat next to Dino. She also had soft, wavy, light brown hair. I could remember turning to look across to her and noticing her strong and determined jaw and lovely caring face. Barbara sat beside her, tall and slim and attractive, with an engaging smile, and Massimo was at the end, dark and handsome and happy, in his white shirt and elegant beige trousers.

How enjoyable the show I'd watched had been! It began with the smallest dancing girls, in fluffy, white, gauze tutus, dainty and petite, flitting backwards and forwards like air-bound fairies in a forest with Titania. Their hair was taken up off their young faces, and wound through with attractive white flowers, which increased the idea of a woodland bower. They were just a tiny bit tentative with their steps at times, but they didn't forget where they were, and caught up easily and naturally. Looking across at Dino's face while they were on, I could see he hadn't expected quite so much involvement from the audience, or that the young girls' routine would be so sweet! He sat completely entranced!

The set was a large, cut-out tree in the middle of the stage. Big, balloon-like shapes filled the branches, white like the rest of the plant, and pretty, multicoloured abstract flowers were painted on. It was a robust set, complimenting perfectly the dancers' outfits, being so strong and sturdy and straight, compared to the see-through, fluffy, wispy skirts at the top of the girls' white, tightly clad legs! The flowers reminded me of enormous smarties, fun and primary coloured – a great contrast to the more intricate and complex real flower arrangements at the front of the stage. Spotlights only illuminated the white of the dancers and the set, and they all achieved a floating quality as they stood out from the black nothingness behind them.

Act had followed upon act for two hours – beautifully differently costumed and cleverly choreographed! The entire audience was very warm and appreciative, not least of all us!

One catchy number used a silhouetted black and silver star and moon backdrop, with dancers clad in rainbow-coloured satin night-shirts, forming a linked row, like a vivid, slinky caterpillar, when they said their goodnights and good mornings at either end of their routine!

And, to finish, the best dancers in the school did a glamorous Arab dance – some wearing dramatic black, leaving a bare midriff to show their accomplished belly dancing to the greatest of effect, and others in demure, white, floaty dresses, using large, flat, grey, leaf fans to cool the air. Stefano, the school's star pupil, leapt high and twirled fast – to our minds nearing perfection – as he courted the beautiful dancing girls around him! Having seen him dance every week I arrived early for my class, in the course before my own, I knew, like all his companions, that his bravura was a combination of talent *and hard work*, and that he and all the girls deserved their rapturous applause!

So it had been... Dino had never seen ballet before, and had been afraid of being bored! When he took me home, I apologised for having half twisted his arm to come and join us! He said he wouldn't have come unless he'd wanted to, and he was so glad he had! That was one of the great things about Dino – I never had to feel guilty that I might have pushed him into things he didn't really want to do, because even if I pressed him, he always took responsibility for his own decisions, having no recriminations for the *'yeses'* and *'noes'* he decided upon. He quietly regulated how much influence from me he'd like in his life, as I supposed I did with him, and we got on with that, leaving each other to get on freely with our doings when the other wasn't around – to see our friends whenever we chose, for example, for just as I trusted him, he trusted me.

Dino still phoned me every week from Italy. Six months apart had seemed at times an infinitely long time. I looked forward very much to his calls. It was so disappointing to have to report time and again that I was too ill with my never-ending flu-like symptoms to be able to go anywhere in England, let alone back to Conegliano, Veneto, and see him again. I just could sometimes hardly bear to think I'd have to wait at least a further couple of debilitated months before I could meet his usually loving self once more!

Would I were fit enough to dance again! In the drier, milder climate of Caserta, where I'd lived for two years with Umberto, one year I'd done a 'keep fit' class twice a week in the early mornings, as then I'd taught English later in the day. I'd drive from Centurano, one side of the busy, bustling town of Caserta, to Casagiove, the other side, and join Sarah and Carmella and Maria for an hour of stretching and toning that was surely extremely necessary after eating the large and extra flavoursome meals of the south!

...Everything had seemed larger than life near Naples, including the food! Enormous plates of pasta and giant vegetables! Large sweet cakes to munch with coffee! In truth, in every way daily existence there for me could take on the exaggeration of street theatre. Generally speaking, I'd flail my arms around more, and become extremely animated and lively, raising my voice, if necessary, with the best, and no doubt sounding at the very least angry and argumentative, whilst merely discussing the prospects of the day!

One year in the south I'd taught at a local grammar school – at first rather reluctantly, as I was trained to teach adults, but I'd enjoyed the challenge of helping with pronunciation, intonation and idiomatic expressions with the four hundred or so students greatly in the end.

The school itself was situated, handily for me, near Caserta, at Maddaloni, a smaller town, bustling and full of traffic in the centre, but peaceful in the outskirts where we were. Near us, behind imposing gates, was an ornate Ducal Palace, now intelligently and effectively used as a boys' orphanage, where the youngsters were brought up and educated by a caring, inspired local priest. The expensive fees paid for sending children to the exclusive private grammar school I taught at were said to be used to enable the care to be provided for the orphan boys.

At Easter and at Christmas, every class from the grammar school would walk, crocodile fashion, quite a sight in their navy uniforms, (rarely used elsewhere in Italy), to the large, spacious courtyard of the Ducal Palace, where row upon row of wooden chairs would be set out, ready for us all to celebrate a solemn mass. We would be preceded by a small, enthusiastic boys' brass band, sent from the orphanage to escort us. The passers-by would stop their round of shopping, and smile benevolently at the sight! After the service, as we filed up to leave, books and Christmas and Easter cakes would be handed to one and all.

Sometimes during the week there I'd have a free hour between lessons, and I could remember one such Tuesday morning. I'd braved the *looks* at a foreign woman going *alone* into a bar, and had matter of factly ordered a cappuccino and gone to sit at a little round wobbly metal table outside! I'd started to read the paper, and then I'd heard clip-clop, clip-clop, from a distance, up the street! In due course some beautiful, glistening black horses had gone slowly and decorously by, poshly dressed in their Italian red, white and green plumes, as well as their shiny, polished black leather harnesses and golden decorations, sparkling in the morning sunlight. Behind them was pulled an elaborate black and gold carriage, and I'd picked up my bag to get my camera out. Then I'd noticed – inside was a coffin, it was a solemn funeral procession.

The sight, as I sat reflectively with my paper, had been so unexpected, and so lovely. There were exquisitely arranged flowers in the regal carriage, and I thought to myself that if it were only for me, I'd have taken that photo! But I remembered Umberto, who every time he saw a black hearse, or a covered black gondola in Venice, would superstitiously hold his small and fore fingers out in the unmistakable shape of two devilish horns, in order to ward off any possible bad influences, and I thought that some of the sad mourners might be equally offended as he would be at a photo being taken, and so I'd desisted.

Umberto, I thought, perhaps too irreverently to myself now as I remembered, had made his two-handed, downward pointing horns *three* times on a single journey one Easter when we'd been travelling from Caserta to Venice to visit his family. He'd been more than horrified to see three funerals on the same trip! He'd been sure it would bring us terrible bad luck. Very fortunately he'd been wrong!

Even when he'd left me, despite everything, I'd been lucky, having a caring family and friends and a good job. I'd been able to make the most of my new-found freedom, even though I'd begged him to give us longer together, so we could try harder. Anyway, it was all in the past now.

I closed my eyes, and knew that I was nearly over Umberto at last – I hadn't had to busily work through more grieving at his loss, only to keep my thoughts as light as possible, and in a miraculous way I was feeling better in my spirit about it all. This realisation made me more hopeful for a recovery from what I had now learned was the illness ME, or post-viral fatigue syndrome – I believed that the burden of past worries and anxieties might have been taking up energy that could otherwise have been directed by my brain towards healing my physical ailments. I prayed that my healing would speed up...

What *could* I do to pass those never-ending hours of rest? I still needed to rest for most of the day, although I was feeling much better when I did get up.

Were there any more light, happy memories of Italy? I looked at a few photos, and the dance cruise came back to me! A *dance cruise*, round the Mediterranean for a week. Even that I'd been lucky enough to do in the summer of '88! Exactly two years ago, twelve months after Umberto had gone, and about three months before I'd met Dino! There were due to be three experienced dance teachers on board, giving masterclasses for the whole week. Classical and modern and jazz teachers were supposed to be coming. We were told that students from dance groups all over Italy would be joining us, and it seemed such a good initiative that I eventually decided to go. I could picture it all so clearly! Only a very small number of young students and their chaperone mothers came from Conegliano in the end – and no one else turned up from the rest of Italy whatsoever! After the big build up, Marta herself had opted for going to America, and didn't even join the cruise. She left that and the final arrangements to her mother!

But those of us who *had* gone, had had a fabulous time! I'd met Davide, as he was a good friend of Marta's mum, and he, along with his close friend Franco, joined me for meals at the same table. The three of us spoke French, and that was very handy, as the only masterclass dance teacher who did finally come was from Paris! She taught classical ballet, and spoke neither a word of Italian, nor of English!

Now I was ill in bed in Ridlow, I thought that that cruise belonged to another lifetime, when I could exercise, and travel, and laugh more loudly without my chest feeling it was going to collapse. I was tired now, and the days all merged together, with little to distinguish one from another. ...Such a wonderful collection of photos had been taken by Davide!

The colours were vibrant in those pictures! I saw the elegant ship *Amelia* docked in Genova, from where we'd left. I remembered our small group amicably sorting out our shared cabins and getting to

know our way around! ...Our first port of call had been sunny
Barcelona, where we'd visited the fine cathedral and the quaint
backstreets, before moving on the next day to dreamy Majorca, where
I'd been lucky enough to see the misty, mysterious Carthusian
monastery where Chopin had come to live with George Sand. The
following day, I was reminded, we'd been to Carthage and the
evocative, ancient ruins that we'd freely explored under a blazing hot
sky... We'd followed on to the very English town of La Valletta in
Malta, where we'd sat by a crowded, uninviting beach for lunch, and
then, I recalled, we'd gone to Siracusa in Sicily, where we'd had an
exceptional guide, and done a lot of sightseeing. I could recall Davide
and I ordering a freshly squeezed refreshing orange juice for our
masterclass teacher and ourselves, and she and I buying some tiny
yellow Sicilian carriages, pulled by minute horses. They had
colourful scenes painted round the sides, and carried a large spare
wheel!

Umberto's father had given me one once, which I'd always
treasured, and I was so happy to be able to get a few more, which
were to be gifts for special people. Finally, on the last day of our
cruise, we'd been to Capri – where I'd so often gone with Umberto
during our years in the south, and I'd taken off alone, walking to the
familiar gardens, to see again the captivating view of the Faraglioni
rocks in the blue sea below. A reminder of what had been...

I looked at the end of the album, and there were some more loose
photographs, showing the impromptu beauty contest on deck, which
I'd forgotten about! There I was, by the swimming pool, as the
entertainment staff had good-naturedly roped me in to entering the
competition! I'd been lying comfortably sunbathing on a deckchair
next to Franco and Davide, on the higher, less crowded, cooler deck,
idly mulling over one or two differences I'd noticed between the north
and south of Italy, which one of the girls had asked me about. I was
thinking about greetings between people who didn't know each other!
How most people I'd met in the north would be formal and polite,
much as in England, saying, "Hello", or "Hello, pleased to meet you"
– and in Caserta how I'd invariably been greeted with, "Hello, how
are you? Are you married? Have you got any children?"!

I'd been interrupted, and whisked off down the steps, with my
dancing companions and about eight more girls. We'd been escorted
one at a time round the four sides of the pool by a burly gentleman in

shorts, who halfway round had stopped and asked what we were looking for in our ideal man! I remembered saying something about a good sense of humour!

We'd sat down patiently in the shade, to await the outcome. I could remember my amazement when I'd been called third! I'd received a little plaque, and there I was in the photo, smiling, surprisingly relaxed, and able to bear all those eyes upon me. All I wanted to do now was hide away, because I couldn't respond to any attention. I sadly had so little energy to give people.

Chapter Seven
July 1990

I felt more cheerful at the beginning of July, and could detect a slight improvement in my energy level! I began to hope I really was finally on the mend. It was so much easier to stay positive when I was stronger. I told myself that I *would* get completely well again one day, and that I should count on it! One day in the summer of '88, I'd been travelling to Venice on a fast train which had come across Europe, feeling rather sad, and for the whole hour journey unusually only one person had sat with me in the non-smoking carriage. Umberto had left a year before, and I was anxious about not perhaps getting enough work, as I'd decided to freelance – I was rather listless and down.

The young, cheerful, athletic-looking, dark-skinned man and I had talked a little about our respective selves for a while – in English, which he spoke almost better than I did, although he was Swiss German! He was a forestry worker and a ski instructor, and told me about the thrill of skiing on fresh powder snow where no one had been. Suddenly he'd changed the subject and asked, "Do you know Stevie Winwood?" 'No,' I'd replied, surprised, "I'm afraid I don't." And as our train drew with increasing power away from Mestre, he'd carefully taken out his small, black walkman and held it to his ear intently for just a moment before handing it to me. "Listen to the words of that song," he'd said "*Back in the High Life again*, – that's you – you'll see that you'll get back to the high life – you think you might not now, but I know that in less time than you think, you*will*. You'll see!"

Lizzie, athletic, slim and attractive, kindly came to visit, and stayed for the usual half an hour, so as not to tire me too much, and was very positive. She was sure I'd get back to teaching by the summer, and be able to do a few courses before returning to

Conegliano for the next academic year, in September. I told her about Steve Winwood's song and she reassured me, "*of course* you'll get back to the high life again!"

Linda came the next day, also for half an hour, and sympathised with me greatly for having been taken away from my life in Italy so suddenly and unexpectedly. She'd met most of my friends there from holidays in both the north and south. She'd learned Italian, and was able to converse and therefore knew them quite well.

It was so hard to make normal conversation, and relate to the world of work that I'd left (I had taught for three years in Cambridge with them) because I had very little news to impart, and my overriding concern was my health, pushing me to be especially interested in it, having almost no energy for anything beyond my daily housebound existence. I longed to tune in again to the vitality and power of having some control over my days, which were all dictated to by how bad or not I was feeling. Sometimes the days seemed endless, but I looked at television in the early evenings with my parents and Granny, and we'd seek to have a laugh wherever one could be gleaned... which helped enormously.

I still had to rest a lot, and invariably my thoughts returned to the Italy I'd left behind. My family and I watched holiday programmes from Italy, Italian opera (softly), Italian cookery... It was great to be able to take it in better by now, despite my migraine-type headaches which plagued me ... and best of all I continued to have many phone calls, cards and letters from my friends and students in Italy, which I had more energy to deal with now, and which kept me in touch with what I was missing. I was still shocked that bad influenza, which is what my illness continued to be like, could carry on for months, and maybe even years, or forever.

In mid-July, with the warmer weather, my mind returned to Caserta, where I'd lived so happily with Umberto for two years. It was such a beautiful, fresh day, I didn't just want to lay on the bed and reminisce... I rolled over, after my afternoon repose, and got up slowly, briefly leaving my Italian thoughts behind and I went to sit outside in the secluded, sweet-smelling garden for half an hour. My fair-skinned mother and grandmother didn't much like the heat from the sun, or the occasional bugs or itchy bites outside, so both were in the cool dining room, chatting, and my father and Rusty were out in the brilliant hot sunshine and breezy shade respectively, lying peacefully and silently on the grass, enjoying the warmth in the air!

I lay flat on a comfortable, albeit creaky lounger, half in the shade and half out, because the glare hurt my eyes, and immediately the bright sun took me back to the time when, years ago, Umberto and I had been living in the hot, dry, healthy climate of Caserta! We were there in the south of Italy because of Umberto's chosen profession, constructing a much-needed aqueduct. We'd rented very reasonable furnished accommodation in a black painted condominium on the outskirts of the military town, with the small rooms cheap and cheerful, and full of what I called matchstick chairs and tables, that looked ready to fall to pieces! That first year we had had, we felt, nothing to entice us to keep indoors at weekends, except perhaps the fascinating horror of the enormous bright brown, round flower heads that positively leapt off the pale kitchen tiles all around you and seemed as if they'd like to come and join you at the table as you sat and ate, because they looked a bit like hedgehogs! Almost without fail, we'd get a couple of fresh ham and cheese rolls together, two cans of lager, some crunchy red Anurche apples, and then take off, and drive anywhere everywhere, all around the exceptionally interesting and thoroughly beautiful region of Campania. We'd loved having our simple picnics, exploring on our own some fabulous settings, which we reached in our intrepid little maroon Lancia Fulvia Coupe!

In Naples, we'd often shop and *window-shop* – one of Umberto's favourite pastimes! We'd also treasured going for a delicious pizza, cooked with love in a wood fire oven. 'Our' pizzeria was busy, bustling, efficient and neatly tucked away upstairs. There was a never-ending camouflage of 'artistic' scaffolding around it! Inside, you forgot all about that as soon as the inviting smells welcomed you and you saw the expertise of the pizza chef! The speciality of the house was a light and tasty, crispy base, with fresh salad tomato, succulent buffalo mozzarella and sweet basil topping!

Thinking of that pizzeria reminded me of a particular day after we'd been going to eat there on and off for about a year. Umberto was truly wonderful about giving me fresh flowers. Each Saturday, almost every week, he'd promptly arrive to pick me up from the grammar school, in the late morning, holding maybe a sturdy, yet delicate-looking, little purple orchid, or a spindly, summery, attractive bunch of broom, or sometimes budding pink or yellow roses, or, in fact, any charming, smallish cut blooms, from the wonderful, rambling, lively Caserta market. He'd always kindly offer the flowers to me with a kiss, before we'd set out on our adventures!

But Umberto absolutely wouldn't buy me any flowers when he felt gently or strongly coerced by someone trying to sell to him! Almost every time we were sitting chatting animatedly in our Neapolitan pizzeria, enjoying our lunch, an elderly, swarthy man would arrive, armed with a large bunch of red roses. "No," he'd firmly be told, if once, then time and time again! Until one Sunday lunchtime he just handed me a single red rose, with a little polite bow, avoiding the usual keenly fought battle of wills, saying huffily that he didn't *want* any money!

My delightful Saturday morning flowers would sit comfortably on the back seat, with their little rounded, plastic water containers on the ends of their stems, or a damp tissue round them, covered in foil, and they would invariably go sightseeing with us! Maybe we'd all go to a picturesque monastery on a steep hillside, or to a crumbling, weathered amphitheatre, a splendid Capodimonte porcelain museum, or to drink in the beauty of small lakes, or spectacular mountains, of winding, tucked away roads up wooded hillsides – or we might go looking for ever splendid and romantic views of Vesuvius, or sometimes leave our car parked in Naples' busy port and take the morning or lunchtime boat over to Capri! There, instead of heading for the handy funicular railway rising up the cliff to the town of Capri, Umberto would head us off at a smart pace up the many steps to the lovely square. I'd never even been *on* that railway!

Out of season, when the tourist traffic wasn't heavy, on a glorious sunny day we'd also love to head for the exceptional Amalfi coast, where the rough cliffs would stand out so clearly and well defined from the blue sea and sky! We'd stroll through the narrow streets and soak up the slower pace of life after our busy weeks in the faster moving town of Caserta. We'd breathe in the sea air and unwind!

We might go along the winding coast from the jewel of Amalfi to the chic and expensive Positano, or make for the equally spectacular beauty of Ravello, perched high on the cliff, with glorious views, where we'd keenly explore wonderful villas and feel ourselves relaxing in the fresh air.

Umberto and I had got on so well that first year in the south. He hadn't been so claustrophobic and his outbursts of temper weren't so bad then as when he returned to northern Italy to be near his family. We'd worked really hard during the week, inspired by the thought of escaping at weekends. In winter months, Umberto and I might often be tempted towards Naples. We'd perhaps make our way through the city to see the beautiful statue of the veiled Christ, finely and serenely carved in white marble, so moving and restful, in the Cappella San Severo. Or on sunnier days occasionally we'd take off for Sorrento, Pompeii, Ercolano, Paestum, Cuma, or the pleasant towns of Salerno, Benevento, Capua...

As I lay in the garden in England, the time I'd previously spent in the south of Italy took on a dreamlike quality, and I believed such colourful memories must be therapeutic – they really helped me feel more positive and alive, and although those days were past, no one could stop the thoughts filling my mind and helping a smile to emerge. How Umberto and I had taken to Campania!

Every now and again we'd like to feel we were following in Virgil's footsteps, when we visited the dark and brooding Lake Averna, for example! I remembered telling Umberto that those mysterious waters were once said to be the entrance to the underworld, as the poor birds flying over would fall in, overcome by the rising noxious gases!

When my family had come to stay near us on the lovely island of Ischia for a week, it was great. Umberto had moved back to work in Asolo in the north of Italy, before I joined him at the end of the academic year, so at that time I was there on my own! My parents and sister had appreciated the island greatly, finding it very beautiful, which made up for the disappointment of finding their hotel rather unwelcoming and overly geared to the many German holidaymakers, with very little English attempted, or spoken.

What a journey I'd had to go and join them for a day! I could remember driving down to Caserta station at top speed in the early morning, and hastily leaving the car, after having been ordered to repark it even closer to the car next to it by the white-capped car park attendant, protecting the cars during the day for just a small fee. I'd hurriedly taken the train to Naples – next going on the underground to the harbour and waiting for a ferry! I'd only relaxed as I travelled smoothly on the water, and upon arriving on the island of Ischia, had done the last leg and taken a bus to the hotel. Three hours! But it was well worth going and meeting my family for a precious afternoon together. We'd had a lovely, long, rambly walk, buying fruit and hazelnut ice creams and frothy cappuccinos and going back to sit round the inviting pool in the early evening sun.

My family had enjoyed the return journey to Caserta with me the following day. They hadn't minded the time spent on the varying modes of transport, and had loved the fast, clean double-decker train we took from Naples! I'd found I hadn't got the car keys anywhere on me when we pulled up at Caserta station, opposite the grand and impressive Royal Palace, and after ordering a taxi home, and then returning with my father to the car park, I found I'd been in such a terrible rush the day before, I'd actually done the unthinkable and left the keys in the car!

Living in Caserta, I'd seen wheels ruthlessly removed from a couple of cars parked outside overnight, and had once heard of a steering wheel and part of an engine being taken from a car locked 'safely' away in a garage! So I was more than thrilled that nobody had investigated the Lancia and driven it away!

That afternoon, after the episode with the car, we'd gone to visit the grand Royal Palace, where my father had also worked during the war. There were still soldiers posted there in some quarters, mostly doing their compulsory military service, and Umberto and I could hear the lilting *Last Post* played every evening as we retired to bed, along with the less tuneful howling from the pack of wild dogs that come dark would roam around the nearby buildings under construction.

My mother, in particular, had been so pleased to see for herself where my father had been posted for a time. We all appreciated the magnificent and ornate rooms so cleverly designed by Luigi Vanvitelli for Charles di Borbone in the style of Versailles! We'd ended up with the spectacle of the large Capodimonte crib, full of so many splendid pieces, from camels to elephants, which was so sadly to be stolen later.

We also loved the spacious gardens, with the long row of stylised pools and fountains, and little fast-flowing waterfalls, statues, green grass and trees, where my father had used to ride his army horses! We were able to take our time absorbing the views, and for my dad it brought his soldier days back to life. Our walk would be punctuated by the odd rest on the side of the fish-filled pools, watching the orange coy carp confidently move about, creating ever-changing patterns of light and shade in the water.

We'd made our way to look at the group of fenced off deer, as our last stop, prepared to spend some time in their company, but we'd immediately and painfully succumbed to what could only be described as *monster* mosquito bites around our ankles, seemingly coming from the long grass, and had instead all slipped away, back to the Royal Palace, out through the large imposing entrance gates, and home for a cup of tea!

Umberto's parents and brother and sister-in-law had enjoyed visiting the Royal Palace too, on their visits to Caserta! I could remember strolling with them through the shady paths to the small Castelluccia, closed now, but built in the same style as the Palace, classically ornate. Every time I'd been to the Palace the sky had seemed perfect – completely blue, just as it was here in England on this lovely day, and, just as there was calm and stillness in the garden here, there was always peace there, away from the bustle of the streets... Except on public holidays! I remembered! The tranquil grounds then would fill to the brim with lively and chatty picnickers, all over the place fathers and sons would energetically play football, and you could hardly move for friendly people spread out on the grass!

Umberto's parents had come to stay with us for a week. His father was from Calabria originally, and he had the dark skin and eyes associated with the region, while his mother was fairer, brown-eyed and slightly more grey than he was – she'd been born in Venice. Both Umberto's mother and her sister were very petite. His father was tremendously easygoing, methodical, and a real gentleman, while his mother was a live wire, full of boundless energy and very sociable.

Although there wasn't much room in the flat I'd really enjoyed having people to stay! Umberto's parents, unused to travelling by car, had loved seeing the sights, especially places connected in some way with their son! Santa Maria Capua Vetere, for example! They'd loved visiting that small and charming town, where Umberto worked, near historic Roman Capua. It helped them imagine better his daily routine.

We saw the evocative remains of the crumbling Roman amphitheatre, which was second in size to the great Colosseum in

Rome, and I remembered Umberto taking a photo of us. His father had since sadly passed away in the summer of '89. None of the rest of his family had been in touch since my illness began, though I'd written short letters and explained why I was unable to get back to Italy for the time being. I wondered if I'd see them again.

Chapter Eight
August 1990

It was difficult for me to recall the many varied happy times in England – they just wouldn't enter my head! Maybe, I wondered to myself, it was because of an unconscious refusal to accept my English life, as I'd been negatively feeling, and still was, that I'd been stuck in Ridlow against my will all this while!

My working life had also been very happy for several years in Cambridge, but all that I could picture at this time were my much-missed students, some of whom I'd known for three and a half years, left behind in Venice, Treviso and Conegliano, in the middle of their courses... without having been able to make provision for someone else taking over, or anything. As time dragged on, I was feeling terrified that most would pass on to new phases in their lives, without me even having had a chance to say goodbye.

The first day of August had dawned and, as at the end of July, I'd pushed myself in frustration to walk out in the fresh air a bit too far. I consequently now felt worse and more tired again. Dino phoned me up, and I was so sorry to have to report that I'd overdone things slightly, and that I was mainly confined to my bed once more, probably for at least a few days. He was so encouraging and patient, but I wished with all my heart I had more cheerful news to report!

Luckily, an hour after the phone call, when I'd recovered my strength, my sister and her husband James popped round, as they did occasionally, and that helped stop me from dwelling too much on my situation. I'd had my sister and brother-in-law to stay with me in Conegliano for their honeymoon in September '88. Fortunately my working schedule then hadn't really got going until October, and it was relatively easy to work round.

I could see my sister now, in my mind, standing near my flat, taller than me, with attractive blonde, naturally wavy hair, and an infectious smile! She had light brown eyes, and a fairer skin than my father and me, and on the tablets she was taking, had needed a shady sun hat – which really suited her. James was tall and dark, and very slim. He had dark-rimmed spectacles, and looked distinguished, despite his youthful appearance.

The three of us had spent a night away, during their honeymoon, I remembered, at my dear friends Massimo and Enrico's house in the mountains. It had been a jolly gathering, and good practice for my translating! In the evening, we'd gone to a family run restaurant, where earthenware plates and a few glistening copper pans lined the walls, and we'd sat at a long, wooden table, undeterred by not always understanding each other! After a selection of pressed hams, the main dish had been locally farmed succulent and tender wild boar, cooked with a special 'Da Giovanni' ingredient, a drop of sweet and fruity home-made grappa di mirtilli! I reflected that I still hadn't become vegetarian, eating meat in company, but I ate a lot less meat at home.

Andrea, James and I had very much enjoyed our short picturesque drives out in the dappled green, sometimes misty hills, and a charming little walk next to some plane trees, along a narrow path by the tiny trickling stream near my flat. We'd 'discovered' on one outing, the fair-sized crazy golf course well hidden amongst the trees near the watermill at Refrontolo, and often while I was working, Andrea and James would enjoy a peaceful stroll to the centre of Conegliano for a look round, perhaps visiting the home of the great artist Cima da Conegliano, where copies of his famous paintings were to be seen, or stopping for a refreshing cappuccino or pear juice!

I couldn't help but think back – that honeymoon visit had been just before I'd met Dino. Like it or not he kept popping into my mind, every day. His kind, handsome face was as yet unknown to me then! I wished he could come and see me now it was August, if I wasn't up to going to Conegliano to see him – but I knew he always looked forward so much to taking his daughter on holiday, and that he needed to wind down from his busy working routine, relaxing on a hot, sandy beach, as he did so much chasing around with his job. He only had two weeks off. Even if he did make a big effort to come to Ridlow, there was nothing I could do to entertain him, I could barely even talk to him for more than half an hour, and he didn't know any English, so in many ways it would be gloomy and dreary and depressing. My parents and Granny hadn't really got the energy to entertain – it wouldn't be fair to ask anything more of them.

Better to wait until I got better, and take things from there!

My mind went back to Andrea and James' honeymoon. It was less emotive. As well as me cooking them some Italian and English dishes, sometimes we'd packed up my wicker picnic basket and eaten outside by the river or up in the hills, or gone for a tasty local pizza, deliciously dribbled over with hot chilli olive oil!

When any of my family had come over to Conegliano, in the evenings we'd invariably plan to get back to Via Ciro early and eat before seven o'clock, but for some reason we found that by the time we'd arrived and I got the table ready and we sorted ourselves out, it was never earlier than eight! Fortunately none of us had difficulty digesting if we ate late, except my poor mother, so on Andrea and James' honeymoon, there was no problem! But I had begun to wonder how in England my mother and grandmother got food *on the table* for six o'clock at the latest! I tried to console myself by reasoning that everything seemed geared to eating later in Italy, the news, for example was on at eight, and the shops stayed open 'til gone seven o'clock – I guessed that when in Rome, it was just as well to conform to patterns of time as anything else!

I remembered Lizzie and Paul and their little son Jamie, going with me to the River Piave for a picnic, just as all my family had done. I recalled how much I'd admired the expertise of Lizzie and Paul, skimming middle-sized round flat pebbles brilliantly across the water, leaving a trail of six or seven circular ripples!

Oh yes... one Saturday morning downstairs from my flat, Sergio had met Lizzie, Paul, Jamie and me in the sunlit car park, and very kindly offered to take us up into the hills to visit the vineyard of a good friend of his, so my visitors could sample and maybe even buy some guaranteed additive-free local wine!

We'd happily accepted his kind invitation, and gone in two cars. There we were warmly welcomed! Glasses of refreshing white prosecco wine were immediately brought out, and crusty, fresh, soft white bread, with long cream chunky strips of delicious, mild, local cheese were swiftly put before us! Not going with the intention of disturbing Sergio's friend for too long, we had nevertheless spent quite a time outside in the warm sun, chatting about different wines and Italy and England! To our right the tied, sprawling vines stretched row upon straight row down the gentle hillside. We'd had a short wander, and Lizzie and Paul had stocked up!

I decided to write a short letter to Maria and Sergio, to find out how they were getting on. I did miss them!

After filling two sides of writing paper, my concentration was going. I stopped, and I was left with the image of Maria and Sergio standing one October day amongst the stationary, expectant crowds lining Conegliano High Street, with Umberto and me, watching for the colourful, costumed procession of the Dama Castellana, the live chess game, to file past! I'd thought so much of the ebullient spectacle, that the following year, when Umberto had left, and Maria and Sergio had opted for not going, having seen it many times before, I'd gone with Barbara and Jill, and we'd not only stayed to see the passing festivities in town, but had also walked in a group up the winding, shady road to the final destination of the participants, the castle, while the flamboyant show was still proceeding down in the square. We'd chosen a good, enviable viewing position, before too many people arrived.

After a wait, the sound of voices had approached, and the winners had filed slowly into the cobbled square. The sun was going down and the scene was romantic, quietly spectacular. I'd wished I could have seen the visiting flag throwers perform, as I'd so enjoyed a similar show once before, at Marostica, and suddenly they all lined up in the dusky twilight and gave an impromptu 'free' display! The rhythm and pace, the twirling and turning and 'floating' of the flags in the air as they were thrown high, or in an arc from one person to another, in such a beautiful setting, was spellbinding! The evening had ended, not there, but with a totally unexpected firework display. It had been wonderful!

I'd tucked away in my mind then and there the wish to get tickets to see the show itself, and at the beginning of October '89, that had been achieved! Some close colleagues from the University had come from Venice to Conegliano, and, after a large and sustaining pasta lunch, we'd sat in the afternoon sun early, missing the parade, in order to choose seats in the front row. It had turned out to be worth it!

The large black and white chessboard proved a good background for the colourful costumes of the participants. Some were richly robed, with dark green or maroon velvet hats, and all the clothes were very sumptuous. Rows of standard bearers stood patiently at the back, separating the square off from the white Accademia theatre, while the absorbing live chess game took place. When it came to the turn of the flag throwers, that was, of course, my sheer delight!

Umberto and I had been to the more famous live chess game in Marostica, a place well known for its succulent cherries, years before! I'd gone back to that small, attractive town, with Linda, on her birthday, in June, when she was over on holiday, trying to recapture the animated scenes and buzzing atmosphere for her by describing how it had been, a little upset I couldn't quite feel as much joy as I'd expected, but glad to revisit and add to the experience with Linda anyway. I'd enjoyed my 'local' show just as much as the one at Marostica, and felt very lucky to be living in Conegliano.

My Italian and English lives made closer contact several times in August 1990, thankfully, through delightful visits from Italian friends. Lizzie and Linda kindly kept coming to see me for half hour or hourly visits from Cambridge, and now Gabriella and Barbara were over from Italy and going to stay ten days with some mutual friends in our village, so I'd be able to see quite a bit of them.

In the middle of August, before Gabriella and Barbara arrived, my ex-colleague from Conegliano, Jill, came from London for a few hours over lunchtime, anxious not to tire me out, on her way to stay with her sister in Norfolk for a couple of weeks. My energy just about permitted me to eat *and* talk at the same time, and it was fantastic to see her, but after a while I had to go and rest, and it was my mother who took her out for a short drive after lunch to see a little of Bury St Edmunds before she departed.

Then, only a few days later, Davide came, with a friend of his, on his (detoured!) way from London to Oxford! It was marvellous to see him too, and he came after lunch and went before tea, so insisting on not putting any of us to the slightest trouble. It was so sad seeing all of them go.

Gabriella and Barbara brought me some baggy white knee-length cotton shorts, and a striped green and orange long-sleeved T-shirt. And I was thrilled! The brightness of the colours and the with-it style seemed to make me feel less Ridlow-bound! I explained that my flu symptoms came back if I did much and they were very understanding. I couldn't accompany them on any visits or excursions, but could manage short chats out in the garden, with Rusty! They simply said I must have been very tired when I got such a terrible illness... and I agreed I was. The girls' English improved and they went to London for a couple of days, and in no time at all the ten days had passed, and the hour had come to say goodbye. Gabriella and Barbara came round, and we took some photos, and they left us with a lovely chickpea dough they had made, to slice thinly and shallow fry. They, and all my friends had such confidence that it was just a question of time before I did get well, it helped me to think that way too! I started homeopathy treatment soon after they left, as well as acupuncture, I cut out sugars and yeasts as much as I could, and took vitamin and mineral supplements to try and build myself up, along with continuing to have plenty of rest, in the hope that if my friends came over again the following year, I'd be much better, if not completely so.

At the very end of the month, Richard came for a day, on his way back from Wales to Conegliano! He'd had a good holiday, exploring the Gower peninsular, and showed me lots of beautiful photos of near where he lived. Only one year ago exactly, Barbara and I had visited him for a weekend, and several of the scenes were familiar. How I wished I could hop into his Fiat Uno with him, and share the drive back! We had such a laugh, and the time flashed by. I was so glad I'd been feeling a bit better than usual on the day he came.

I was left with a sense of loss after Richard went, at the end of August, because I'd secretly counted on being fit again by then, and being able to return to Italy and see everybody, starting a new academic year. I just didn't know now if I'd ever get better.

I went to look at a couple of photos Richard had taken and once given me. They were snapped in the mountains, at Nevegal, an hour away from Conegliano, and the snowy scenes soothed me. I wanted so desperately to believe that one day a high life returning would allow me to spend time doing things in company with my friends again! But... skiing, would I ever be fit enough to ski again?

I had to laugh to myself – I would always be a hopeless skier, but the peace and beauty and majesty of the snow-covered peaks and coniferous trees against a blue sky couldn't but inspire anyone! Although I'd never been drawn to the cold weather, and hadn't much liked winter before moving to Conegliano, I'd been fortunate enough to discover that if you dressed appropriately and snugly, it could be *fun!*

When I'd gone skiing with Richard and his other friends in his car, I'd loved opening the door to the first rush of cold, crisp air, and getting out on to the glistening, hard-packed tracks of ice, avoiding the slushy, wet, muddy areas, where many people had passed...

Barbara and Richard and Giuliano had got on with skiing faster than me, and so while they tested their skills on more challenging *pistes*, I'd potter slowly about on the beginner and intermediate slopes! We'd all make a rendezvous at lunchtime, and sit out at wooden tables catching up on how we'd done. Jill came too sometimes, and went for an invigorating walk surrounded by the beautiful mountains, as she had yet to learn to ski. We'd generally leave early, while many people were still skiing, to avoid the traffic jams on the way back, and it could be quite a relief to take my tight-fitting ski boots off and relax my feet. How I loved those mountains!

Chapter Nine
September 1990

September came – this year would it be my favourite month? Could I keep hold of Italy in my mind, or would I forget it? I was in a quandary. I had to start letting memories go, instead of clinging to them, but I didn't want to! September in the Veneto, where I used to live... Oh to be there for the *Festa dell'Uva*, the wine festival, and the tail end of the Venice Lido *Leone D'Oro* film festival, before working life got really hectic again in October! Generally speaking the weather was not so cloying or humid as it could be in July and August, and there was a plethora of lovely fresh sunny days to *get out and about* in!

September 24th 1990, in Ridlow; I was still in bed, after not having picked up greatly from overdoing things, and I *reluctantly* celebrated my thirty-fourth birthday for the most part flat on my back again. My understanding mother, who'd gradually comprehended my illness better over the past nine months, kindly put some pretty pale pinks and dainty gypsophila in a small green vase on the side near the door in my room, and I had some lovely yellow roses from Italy, from Dino. Philip, my homeopathic and acupuncture practitioner thoughtfully gave me a charming bunch of shaggy, unusual, large-headed chrysanthemums, which also made the room feel fresher and lighter, so I was very lucky. I briefly reflected – rather wryly – that it was a good job Umberto couldn't see the chrysanthemums inside the house, for he'd believed those particular flowers were only for taking to cemeteries, and that inside a home they'd bring terrible bad luck!

I was fortunate enough to have some useful presents, including a new V-neck cream jumper, which seemed perfect for the autumn. I was looking forward to getting up and wearing it.

Not many people knew the date of my birthday, I'd thought, and I'd been surprised and delighted with my thirteen cards! They'd had the effect of greatly cheering up both my bedroom and me! It was so nice not to feel forgotten. I was also thrilled to receive eight telephone calls. I felt contact with the world at large a bit more, and really positive by the end of the day!

On my birthday, I didn't feel well enough to go to Philip's Aberdey Clinic in Newmarket, and instead, as I was so poorly, Philip generously came round and gave me some more homeopathic remedies at home. They relieved the limpness and the acute aches a little. Although progress with the treatment was slow, it nevertheless was almost imperceptibly felt each time, and I believed it was like building with blocks, which one day I'd be able to kick away from underneath me when I reached the platform of good health I was aiming for. It was as if I'd fallen off that platform of good health, as I'd got so ill so suddenly, and I'd ended up right down to near the bottom of a gully, on Christmas Day 1989, when my pneumonia had started so severely! Anything was better than nothing, however painstaking, and I was simply too weak for acupuncture, and very grateful for Philip slightly relieving the pain and bringing about my gradual improvement through using homeopathic tissue salts, vitamins, minerals, extraction remedies, essential oils and Bach flowers. I was more tired while I felt the treatments working but, possibly thanks to them, was able to go downstairs and face some television programmes with my family by the evening.

During the whole of my birthday I couldn't help but think of Dino, and wonder whether we'd have spent the evening together! Perhaps we'd have gone to a favourite restaurant of his in the hills, and to the piano bar later, to listen to some music? Or maybe I'd have cooked an early evening meal, and we' d have stayed in?

It was exactly two years ago that Dino and I had met – at the beautifully situated outdoor swimming pool, at San Pietro di Feletto, nestling in the Veneto hills! I smiled to myself as I remembered... I'd been lying on the warm concrete, close to the edge of the children's pool, hearing the lively chatter around me without concentrating on it, whilst relaxing comfortably – after sorting out autumn course timetables! Dino had been there, with several younger friends, who at one stage had taken turns to push each other effectively into the main pool! There had been a young, attractive girl of about eight playing near them, who looked very like Dino, and he'd been so attentive during the afternoon, teasing her and getting ice-cream and drinks, that I'd wondered if he was divorced, and looking after his daughter with his friends for the day.

As the play-acting had lost momentum, the group had all settled down again quietly, but I could see that Dino was a bit fidgety and bored. In the end, after about half an hour, he'd come up and sat beside me, and asked if I could be pushed in! I'd pleaded for my watch, and we'd sat happily, dangling our legs and feet in the tepid water of the shallow pool, talking at length about the world and ourselves, and liking each other! I'd been going out with my good friend Giovanni for about six months during the fifteen months since Umberto had gone, but he'd been so busy, and away a lot, not bothered about a strong commitment, that things hadn't really worked out, and so although we'd been very in tune to start with, we'd stopped seeing each other in June.

Dino had asked me out that first time we met, but I'd been a bit cautious, saying I'd think about it! I didn't want to rush into anything. He said he often went to the pool, so I knew where I could find him! I hadn't had to, as it turned out, because a few days later, as I was crossing the road back to my flat, with both hands holding large plastic carrier bags full of fruit and vegetables, his car had pretended to run me over, and he'd leaned out of the window and asked me to go for a drink that evening! I'd thought I might as well say yes!

I thought back to my birthday a year ago, and on this very same day in '89, at this time, Dino and Jill and I had been walking round the centre of Conegliano, enjoying the wine festival. Small wooden boxes of sweet dessert Moscato grapes, and a few of uva fragola– the distinctive, small, round, purple strawberry grape – were being sold in the main square, eye-catchingly tied with red ribbons over the cellophane; and in the covered, arcaded corner of the piazza, cream ceramic carafes, with Conegliano Castle hand drawn in blue and brown on them, were on sale next to the outdoor chessboard! Red, white and sparkling local wines could be bought by the glass or the bottle from behind long trestle tables, and there was a friendly, harmonious atmosphere!

There was even a large, pink and white striped hot-air balloon, anchored in the square, with a basket large enough to pop four children in underneath it, taking them up as high as the top of the Accademia theatre, and down again!

In the evening, at about six thirty, Richard and Giuliano had joined us, and we'd all gone up into the hills to one of our favourite restaurants, Alla Sorte, for a lovely 'birthday' meal. It was Giuliano's birthday the day before mine, so over the years, we'd taken to having a joint celebration. Dino still didn't know my other friends very well, so it was a good opportunity for them to get together! He looked smart in his pale beige trousers, which he'd put on instead of his usual jeans, and he was particularly quiet that evening, no doubt weighing things up. The next day he told me how much he'd enjoyed the meal, and that he'd not said much, as he'd been afraid of showing me up, having left school at fourteen! Which was, of course, ridiculous!

The hills had been bathed in moonlight as we'd come down from the restaurant, and it had been very romantic. I'd been with Dino in his car, and I had noticed that he seemed a little more relaxed when we were on our own!

I thought about Alla Sorte, where Jill or Richard or Barbara and I would sometimes go to lunch at the weekends. Then, instead of sitting inside, we'd get a round table under the trees, and a carafe of house prosecco would miraculously appear before us as we sat down! Water would eventually join it, and we'd tuck in to soft white bread and crisp grissini, while awaiting to hear the menu. This was very seasonal, which was marvellous, and it was comprehensive, changing all the time! Usually we'd go to Alla Sorte by car, but Jill and I had walked the two and a half miles there once, and appreciated our lunch even more!

It was truly such a joy driving through the hills round Conegliano. I'd often go for a walk with Richard on a Saturday afternoon, and on the way we'd soak in the beauty of the scenery. I could remember us stopping one day when we'd seen a sign for honey at the side of the road – we'd gone in, and found that some clear, chestnut honey was for sale, which the lady told us was particularly good for asthma and bronchial trouble. I'd bought some immediately. I even missed that half-empty jar!

During the warmer months, Giuliano and Richard and Barbara and I would often go for walks at weekends which really blew the cobwebs away! I looked forward to them all the week. We'd usually go to the hills, and had had great fun last year watching hang-gliders systematically prepare themselves for take off, moving back away from the edge of a large, steep, flat-topped hill that fell right away to one side, and running forward towards it, safely harnessed to their wings, and jumping off into space in front of our noses, floating away. My two friends Riccardo and Massimo had done a hang-gliding course for a year once, and they assured me that the terror of leaping out into nothing had never got better, and that fascinating as it might look, if I was dubious even about skiing, then it probably wouldn't be the sport for me! They didn't have to convince me! I hadn't the slightest wish to try it myself, although I admired and loved watching other gallant people who enjoyed it take off.

Richard and Giuliano were wonderful companions on Sunday afternoons sometimes too. We'd split up around six o'clock, and they'd usually meet other friends in the evening, often in Treviso, while I'd spend the time with Dino, after his football match, once he'd taken his daughter back to her mum for the week. Invariably I'd be called for in the early afternoon by Richard and Giuliano, and Giuliano would drive us to some rejuvenating and heart-warming destination in his Fiat Uno – which was deep blue, and just the colour I'd have chosen, given the choice! One or the other always drove, which I was so grateful to them for, as they knew that freelancing I had an extremely tiring week, commuting backwards and forwards to Venice and Treviso, and they were real gentlemen!

My most poignant of many cherished memories of outings together was of one just before I'd come back to England for Christmas in '89. I'd already got the recurring flu, though at that stage I'd seemed to be getting over it, and Richard and Giuliano had carefully bundled me into the back of the car, instead of leaving me on my own, stuck inside the flat, where I'd been all the morning resting, on a beautiful warm, sunny afternoon. Rather than go for a walk, which I hadn't felt up to doing, they'd suggested we drive to a little place called Sarmede, where there was an international exhibition of children's book illustrations! I'd secretly been feeling so achy and rough that I hadn't envisaged going anywhere at all, and I'd been so touched that Richard and Giuliano had included me in their outing, which brought me such joy!

We'd loved the imagination and variety of the fascinating exhibition, which I'd never heard of before. It wasn't enormous, and just right for me to look round without feeling exhausted. One painting of a castle ramparts and moonlit courtyard, with an open book lying forgotten on the ground, had taken my eye straightaway, and, after a short browse, I'd gone to see if there were any posters of it for sale. There were, and I'd splashed out and bought two! One for Linda, and one as a souvenir, which I rarely did, for myself! It had seemed so ethereal in the blue-tinged moonlight, and romantic, as though a young princess had been reading alone to pass the time, and had absentmindedly dropped the book when her Prince Charming had unexpectedly arrived, and swept her gallantly away in his arms!

About to go to sleep after a surprisingly happy birthday in Ridlow, still ill, some vague persistent thought came back to me about having once been told that I myself would meet a knight in shining armour! I tried to place where I'd heard that, in what context, and in a few minutes it clearly came back to me!

It was on a train journey, from Naples to Venice, with Barbara, and her Sicilian mother. They'd started their journey in Palermo, and Umberto and I had bumped into them as we'd got on. That was how we'd met in the first place. After a while, Barbara's mother had taken out a pack of Sicilian tarot cards, and to help pass the time, had told Umberto and I our fortunes. They'd assured us it was very light-hearted – there was no card of death, for example, and the predictions mainly consisted of whether money was to shortly come to you, a journey would perhaps take place, a serious talk with someone might materialise, and so on! We'd taken everything with a pinch of salt, and become good friends in eight hours. Barbara's mother had told me I'd meet a knight in shining armour, and I'd thought she'd got the tense wrong, and that it was Umberto.

When Umberto and I had met Barbara and her lively, friendly mother, we'd been travelling to Venice for a long weekend, to see the popular carnival! The unique alleyways and splendid squares lent themselves so well to people walking about or posing in costume – traditional and modern! It had been a 'cheer myself up' (Tiramisu) weekend, as only six days earlier, Umberto and I had unfortunately been involved in a head-on car crash in Naples, and I'd been mildly concussed. Fortunately nobody had been seriously hurt, and only the other car had been travelling at speed – we'd been slowly turning from a side-street onto the main road by the harbour, and the overtaking car hadn't seen us in the sheeting rain. I still hadn't felt quite back to normal during the train journey, but over the course of the weekend, I'd lost the strange sensation of my brain floating about!

I finished my birthday by thinking about the Conegliano costumes and floats during the wine festival. The Venetian costumes reminded me of Umberto, the Conegliano ones reminded me of Dino. Two green grape-covered floats, variously costumed men and women around them, just flowed into my mind, as I was drifting off to sleep. The first had a *very* large, green grape-covered bottle on it, and next to it a gigantic green grape-covered carafe, with an enormous green grape covered goblet beside it! At the main square the float had halted, and the bottle had sprung into action, after creaking and groaning admirably for a minute or two, slowly tipping the presumed local prosecco into the slightly smaller carafe! Once the bottle had righted itself carefully, the carafe then also tilted over and visibly poured the wine into the waiting goblet. We'd been so impressed! We thought it definitely should have won first prize, though sadly it didn't. The last thing I was aware of was the second float – of human size green grape footballers, called 'Italia '90'! As I'd watched Dino play football a fair bit, I could certainly empathise with his wish to see Italy do well in the forthcoming World Cup! He had squeezed my shoulders when that float went past, and told me that he hoped England would do well too. I'd thought he was teasing me, but he'd been serious!

Chapter Ten
October 1990

As October arrived, I was able to get up again most days, despite the pain still being in my limbs and muzzy head to a certain extent. In the mornings, I'd often go down and sit in the dining room, in a soft chair that didn't press hard on my tender lungs from the back, and have a quiet chat with Granny, or summon up the concentration to read a few short, reasonably interesting articles in her paper! My vision would blur as I focused on the page, on and off, and I almost constantly had a bad head, but it was an improvement from being isolated in my woodland glade, and my hopes of full recovery were high again!

Sometimes Granny would tell me about her first love George, and then her husband John, who'd sadly died thirty-three years ago, when I was six months old. Granny'd always worked hard, and missed her independence and little flat in Ipswich which she'd managed until she was eighty-two. She'd then come to live with my parents, thinking it was best to do so before she got too elderly and infirm. I'd talk in turn with Granny about Venice, because she had met Umberto's family when they'd come over to our wedding, and it wasn't too boring for her if she could picture people she knew! Sharing some of my Venetian memories helped to while away the time happily for the both of us.

I had to admit, that though many early experiences of my life in Venice had been with Umberto, I'd continued going there regularly from Conegliano once he'd gone, and had had equally good times, and I'd had a wonderful month and a half there before I even met him– so it was definitely 'my' place too! …And as I thought back, I suddenly laughed, as I remembered Fred, whom I'd met when I'd first arrived!

I'd encountered this fresh, ruddy-faced, healthy-looking man, with a shock of light blond hair in the departure lounge in England, and strangely enough he'd had the seat next to me on the plane! He had twinkly light blue eyes, and a kind face – he was, I'd guessed, about ten years older than me.

He'd pulled out a thick wad of lira to show me that he'd made his fortune in the building trade, and said he went to Venice every month for a few days, on business. He'd said he was financially very wealthy and would I marry him? He wasn't joking!

I'd talked amicably with Fred during the whole flight, once he'd accepted my 'No!', and eventually he'd relaxed, and accepted we could be friends if he would like, and asked me to do him the honour of dining with him that evening, as he was not starting work until the following morning. I had lodgings in a pension to go to, but knew no one in Venice as yet, so I'd been pleased to agree. We seemed to have little in common really, but it was nice for both of us to have company! We'd gone to a restaurant near St Mark's Square by water taxi – as Fred had too much money, he said, to use public transport!

The meal had been delicious. The restaurant had red awnings in the windows and had tempted us in. Fred had never been there before. During the evening, we'd got on well. Fred hadn't asked me to marry him again! I was relieved, for although he was very personable, I wasn't exactly attracted to him!

Fred had been so good as to see me back to my pension, and then he'd sheepishly admitted he hadn't booked a hotel for himself. He'd asked if he could share my room, as there were two beds – for a night. I'd said 'No', immediately, but had then looked at his tired face and seen his weariness, recognised it was late to go off into the night, and somehow knew I could trust him – and so finally I'd cautiously agreed.

I'd awoken in the morning, to find Fred gone, and a large shopping bag on the side, with milk, biscuits, fruit, sweets, and so on in – with a brief note thanking me, offering me breakfast, and saying goodbye! I'd never seen or heard from him again!

A couple of months later, I'd met Umberto, a pupil at my school, in a friend's class. We'd both had to walk for about half an hour, back to the train station after the evening courses, and had soon got to know each other better, and become close. I had gone on to participate in a lot of Venetian festivities with the joy of seeing them also through his and his kind family's eyes! Carnival, for example, was inextricably linked in my mind with his mother's wonderful round fruit and pine nut doughnuts, along with the 'crostoli', the crunchy traditional biscuits!

Walking round the city, admiring the carnival costumes during that couple of weeks each year had been exciting, and Umberto and I would grab our cameras and try and go out and take the best atmospheric pictures we could! We'd aim to capture the contrast between the people and the place, that both seemed to show themselves off so well, and act a role, but one was static and the other constantly changing. When we walked back from St Mark's Square, via Rialto, we'd always go Umberto's 'special' way, avoiding crowds of people, and the crush!

I was made very welcome by Umberto's parents if I was asked by Umberto to come and stay at carnival time! Should there be flooding, too, his family would immediately lend me a pair of their wellingtons, and I'd be advised where the higher and lower areas of water were, so I could avoid the deeper parts, and not have water go over the top of the boots! Once Umberto had had to put his dark brown thigh length waders on and carry me across about fifteen yards of invading lagoon, which was stopping me from reaching his house!

My mother came in with some coffee for Granny, and so we sat quietly while she drank it. It had Sanatogen nerve tonic in, which Granny swore did wonders for her. She said she always got much more anxious if she forgot to put it in! She had a couple of tasty, crumbly, little cheesy biscuits, as having gone off sweet things, and liking something to 'mop up her coffee', as she put it, they seemed to be ideal! She'd loved it when I had been able to make cappuccinos on the noisy coffee-making machine, and I hoped that one day soon I'd be well enough to stand the ear battering of the milk frother working once more, and make some for her and the rest of the family!

Granny had been very active all her working life, and took an avid interest in what was going on in the world! She conscientiously read through the paper every day, and watched the main evening news at six o'clock, and at nine o'clock, and often at ten o'clock as well! She'd point out anything to me she thought I might find worth looking at, especially if there was anything about ME.

I drew Granny's attention to the fact that Rusty'd brought some little apples in. "What do you mean, Rusty's prattling?" said Granny. And I explained, hoping I wouldn't have to repeat it for the inevitable second or even third time, that Rusty'd picked them up, filling her cheeks to bulging with them, as they'd fallen off the tree. "What do you mean, she's calling out to me?" she'd replied. "I can't hear her! What are you talking about?"

After explaining a second time, as slowly and patiently as I could, I went up for a rest, and lay quietly for half an hour before going downstairs again. This time, images came to me, rather more than events, and it was like suddenly coming across an unexpected mosaic of Venice, sparkling in sunshine, and taking my mind back to intensely happy times, enriching me! I wished Umberto well in my mind, and hoped that one day he'd find what he was looking for, leave his claustrophobia behind, and feel fulfilled.

I had a clear picture of him standing on the Accademia Bridge next to me, watching the Vogalunga, the rowing marathon, pass down the Grand Canal, to the cheers of the many spectators! There were small yet sturdy craft, and large heavy boats with maybe eight or ten fit oarsmen or women in, old and young – and the view out to the rippling lagoon, with so much positive energy being created along the Grand Canal just beneath us – was a sight for sore eyes! The wooden Accademia Bridge was my favourite viewing place, as there was the beautiful, white, harmoniously rounded form of the church of the Madonna della Salute in the background.

The Historical Regatta too came into my thoughts, when Umberto and I had been terribly in love. I could see us sitting on Umberto's brother and sister-in-law's little black dingy, alongside hundreds of other small vessels of all shapes and sizes, moored near the end of the canal, bobbing about on the water as boats passed us – first the historical procession, with the grand, colourful and ornate gondolas and larger boats carrying the costumed Doge in his distinctive hat and his splendidly dressed entourage, and then the racing crew throughout the afternoon! We'd all taken some drinks and biscuits to keep us going, but after a couple of hours, an ice cream was suggested, and quick as a flash Umberto had skipped across the three or four deep boats to the path, more sure-footed at speed than even a young mountain goat! He'd been back very soon, no hands free in case he stumbled, and rejoined us, hopping over people and things as if it were second nature. How we'd all really enjoyed those ice creams!

Then there was the Festa della Madonna della Salute, that he'd shown me my first year, where a bridge of boats was built over the Grand Canal, especially for the occasion, so that people could come easily and pay their respects to the Virgin Mary, thanking her for saving them from the plague. Outside the church, very large, and smaller candles would be on sale, and also nuts in crunchy candy, on little stalls. Inside, generally, every year I'd visited, there'd be choirs singing melodiously, and, despite the enormous space within the church and the many visitors, a real and abiding sense of peace was found.

There were so many wonderful aspects to life in Venice, and I could picture many lively and varied scenes, mostly with Umberto and his family – and then myself, finally, standing at Conegliano station in the early morning, waiting for the train to take me into Venice for work. I always looked forward to arriving, although I preferred to actually live in the country in Conegliano, where I could drive, and feel less cut off from the rest of Italy!

I went downstairs to see Granny again, and my mother had just come back from helping one of our friendly, elderly neighbours put her electricity back on, as she had tripped the switch and been unable to make herself any lunch. My mother was due to go round and see my sister fairly soon after we'd eaten, and take her her prize of honeysuckle talc and soap that Andrea had won at a village coffee morning church draw! I heard about it from my mother who'd been there, and how some kind people had asked after me. There had been home-made cakes on sale, one of which she'd come home with, and about forty pounds had been raised for church funds!

My father came in then from the garden, where he had been working all the morning, among other things clearing up some of the tiny little green apples, that had fallen all over the front lawn. He'd been for his regular morning walk and had met three other people walking dogs. Rusty, by all accounts, had had a great time greeting them all.

Generally speaking, Rusty loved to carry something in her mouth, and she'd often see a stick as she was walking past a hedgerow and carry it all the way round, until she saw another dog, of course, and went to say hello! She might drop it then and we'd think she'd forgotten all about it, but she'd go straight back to it on the way home, and carry it proudly right to the garden, as pleased as punch, where she'd proceed to chew it up! My father was the one who usually went round after her, clearing the heaps of splintery remains away. She'd bring stones back too, and we had quite a pile in the back garden. The more chalky ones she'd even manage to crunch up, to our amazement, and my father and I wished we had teeth as strong as that!

We sat down to lunch. For most of the time since my illness, I hadn't been able to manage sitting on my usual childhood kitchen stool, as there was no support for my back, and after a few minutes I'd feel physically tired and my chest would start to ache. Granny liked to eat in the dining room sometimes, in her chair by the window, with her food on a tray, and I joined her, until the day might arrive when my lungs no longer hurt. I had a fairly good appetite, thankfully, and was very grateful for being so well looked after. I just hadn't myself got the strength to start cooking something like a roast lunch, and if I'd lived on my own, I'd have had to pop a prepared dish into the oven, hopefully – from our exceptionally well-stocked local shop, or one of the handy supermarkets nearby, if I could get there, or ask a kind person to go for me. I wouldn't have been able to make the gravy, then stand and stir it, probably, and my head wouldn't have been able to get round the organisation of cooking times, so that everything was ready together!

I wished I could go out with Rusty and my father for their regular afternoon walk. Once again we were lucky with a day of sunny, warm weather. They would go, I knew, through the grassy footpaths, with rambling, blackberry covered hedges to the left, and dull, golden stubble fields stretching away to the right, as far as the village green, and then either turn right past the peaceful, well-tended cemetery, round by the church, or left past the post office, along the pavements through the village.

I did love Ridlow for its great walks. Just ten minutes away from our house, there was a charming view over the undulating patchwork of fields, full of soft browns, and beiges and greens. We'd always stop and breathe in that scene, as the hues changed with the seasons, and we'd feel refreshed as we passed, occasionally noticing, far in the distance, a small train, shimmering along. I could get as far as that and back very very occasionally, on exceptionally good days.

I often went to sleep at night, dreaming of the view that must have been impressed on my subconscious, from the platform of Conegliano station, which I'd used to see every time I was waiting for the train to Venice! I could see through to the delightful town, where I felt so at home, and a touch of sadness came over me. I had to face the fact that I hadn't got back there for the next academic year, and the knowledge became very real to me that I might have to, unwillingly, kiss my Italian life goodbye, and come to terms with selling up and living indefinitely in England!

Chapter Eleven
November 1990

Christmas was fast approaching, and I was terrified of catching another flu on top of what I had already. Granny was petrified of getting any winter illness as well, believing she was too old and weak to throw it off easily, so we stayed in the house, and effectively 'hibernated', making a right pair! The cold air made it considerably harder for me to breathe, so, on the whole I was glad enough to stay indoors, and as the month of November progressed, my health got distinctly better once more, and I was hopeful yet again of a complete recovery!

If only... If only I had some positive, concrete news about an improvement in my health to write on my Christmas cards to friends in Italy, but there was no way of knowing how 1991 would be for sure. I wrote short greetings on a few cards each day, so as not to get too tired, and I found I was really looking forward to hearing from my dear friends and students more than I ever had in my life before.

Granny loved a blazing coal fire, and, after lunch, we'd light one in the lounge, and all gravitate towards it, as it was soon the warmest room in the house! I'd go in there to write instead of the dining room, still with my several layers of warm clothing on, topped off by a cosy woollen jumper. I had poor circulation and sitting around a lot all day meant I could get very cold. Granny got even colder, and every now and again her right hand would seize in a cramp, while she was doing her tapestry, and I'd have to get up and rub it hard for her. Even doing that small thing soon made my arm ache, and caused me to feel tired – so sometimes I'd have to sit down for five minutes, before finding the energy to rub some more!

Rusty was a great source of comfort, coming in for her cake or sandwich titbits after tea, and stretching out comfortably in front of the fire – if ever she was allowed to! Granny would sometimes shout at her, "Get out of the way dog, you're taking up all the heat from the fire! Go on! Out of the way!" And my father'd say, "She's got a name, haven't you, Rusty dear! She's not doing any harm. She'll move in a minute." And my mother would usually take her mother's side, and eventually Rusty would be banished to 'her' cooler sofa under the window, where she'd stretch out happily again, and my father would go with her and stroke her for a long time!

I was aware I could bear 'to *be* in and *think* England' now, a great deal better than nearly a year ago, when I had felt so forced to be here against my will - there was no doubt about it!

Thoughts of Italy still comforted me though. There was Barbara's isolated, beautiful house in the hills, for example, near Conegliano. I'd been with her and her mother on an exploratory trip to look for a suitably appealing place that could be done up. We'd soon discovered several properties that looked encouraging, and since I'd been in England, they'd eventually settled on a very fine one, which I hadn't seen. Barbara and her mother were hoping I'd soon be well enough to go and stay there. And they were kind enough to say I'd be welcome for months, to convalesce, if I'd like to. ...Would that I could! I recognised that I still wasn't up to satisfactorily looking after myself without a great deal of difficulty!

Barbara's house beckoned me back, as did friends, students... and I longed to see Dino's face again, certain now that if I couldn't return to Conegliano, our relationship would most likely move on no further. Dino still phoned every week, with love, but I couldn't picture him struggling to learn English, and leaving his daughter who needed to have him around, or his stalwart lifelong friends, and challenging, interesting job, without knowing me better before he took that risk. He'd been deeply hurt by his wife leaving him, and he would be devastated should he give up everything he held dear, except for me, and have things not work out between us.

It was no good - however close we were, we simply weren't ready as a couple for him to take such a big step! I wouldn't even ask him to, because I also needed more time to get to know him and love him before I could take on that responsibility. We were both still getting over our past - we'd made slow, painful strides at overcoming that, and I believed that if we'd been granted another year or two before my ME had struck, we'd have very likely decided to be together in

England. I told myself that if Dino and I were *meant* to have a future as a couple, then somehow we would!

So some of the times Dino and I had spent together would now come into my mind, and I'd try and sense what our future would be by letting my mind go blank if I could manage it, then introducing a thought of him, and seeing what sensation I was left with. I always, without fail, got a good feeling, which was reassuring, and I hoped that whatever happened... well, being so ill, and fragile, it was hard to think about!

I could picture Dino and I near my Conegliano home last autumn, at the small, secluded riverbank where he loved to go and fish, and how he'd animatedly and youthfully showed me his four different rods, before we were distracted by the intermittent sounds of cheering and shouting in the background. It had been a rare and much-cherished Saturday afternoon together! We'd investigated the noises, and soon come across an energetic pony race that seemed to be in full swing! Young riders on ponies had been galloping enthusiastically and competitively round a circuit, and were being timed and encouraged as they went. Dino and I had joined the involved spectators for a while, holding hands and feeling for each participant! I'd half wished then that we could spend more such lovely, relaxing weekends together – that he might give up his football commitments one day – and the irony was that only a month after I'd got ill, he'd sadly twisted his knee in a match, and no treatment he had undergone had helped it right itself completely. Whilst it didn't hurt him at all in everyday movement, he couldn't play football, or the pain would come back... and, poor Dino, my half wish had been granted belatedly once I'd gone, he'd given up the game. Almost every Sunday had been free!

That Saturday last autumn had been great, I recalled, because in the evening we'd gone out for a pizza to a flashy place he knew of in Vittorio Veneto – painted in dark purple, with spooky lighting, it nevertheless lived up to its promise of offering one of the most delicious pizzas ever! Dino had ordered for me; a vegetarian one, and it had come topped with super pre-cooked char-grilled aubergines and courgettes, onions, artichokes, peppers, and peas! I still wasn't more than half vegetarian, but by then felt comfortable to be moving in that direction, without guilt, knowing that it would happen when I was ready! We'd had a wonderful time that evening, laughed a lot, shared more of our inner selves, and I was warmed now and comforted by those memories as I lay in bed in Ridlow.

I marvelled that nothing good in life was ever wasted, for happy times in the past were constantly giving me strength to keep positive and hopeful, and courage to persevere with treatments and remedies and a high protein diet and rest and anything and everything that might help me get back to what some people had told me must have been too stressful if I'd got so ill, my old way of life – as a well person! I prayed that I'd once again live my life at that fast pace and intensity! I knew the cause of my illness was just bad luck, or God's will, and that it had hit me so badly because I had been so tired. That was all!

I was sure my friends were right! I'd been mentally exhausted from doing months of extra demanding creative work, on top of my busy schedule, as a favour for a friend, and not wanting to let him down by saying no when I should have done! I'd been emotionally tired by family commitments all the years my sister had been unwell, and getting over Umberto and his family and so on. I'd also been spiritually weary, feeling far away from God, whom I nevertheless believed was within me and without – I'd been doing a lot of interesting but tiring bible study. And least of all, but perhaps with slight significance, I'd been physically tired by adhering to my strenuous weekly jazz dance and squash matches – so I'd had very little resistance when the illness had struck! If I'd caught the flu and ME only a couple of weeks later, I'd have had a fortnight resting behind me, over Christmas, and my tiredness would have been far less pronounced... I felt it wasn't that I'd got ME because I couldn't cope with stress! Stress surely makes things worse, it doesn't cause them to arrive in the first place! ...It was just one of those things!

As November progressed I was glad my growing awareness of England and all things English was growing. It was so painful to have my head mostly somewhere that my body could not be. I began to feel less strange and distant from my family and Linda and Lizzie. I was concentrating more on the present, but a weekend break in Liguria kept coming back to me. The five towns on the coast near Levanto, which had been so enchanting! I'd always longed to see them, ever since Umberto had been, after we'd separated, and he'd told me how charming and pretty they were! I'd gone with Richard, Giuliano, and Barbara, in Richard's car, and we'd called in to see Jill on the way, for she had moved to Mantova! We'd stayed in a spotless pension near the pebbly beach in Levanto, and done a lot of wonderful coastal walking for a couple of days! I'd been so thrilled to see and touch and smell again the dusty green olive trees and awkward prickly pears and bright, startlingly pink bougainvillaea, which I'd missed seeing so much from when I'd lived in the south of Italy!

As we'd walked steadily along well-trodden wide and narrow paths, clambering through woods and out into the full sunshine or cooler, cloudy weather, invigorated by the fresh sea air, we'd seen glorious views of the sea and cliffs and captivating coastal towns below. I'd thought that if ever one day I had the means or the will to buy a second house like Barbara had done, then it would be in the five towns we visited! And I'd forgotten that pesto was a Ligurian speciality, and so had been happily surprised to eat it both evenings we were there.

I found I couldn't concentrate on the beauty of the photos of Liguria when I got them out, because the frustration of my situation was too strong! I put them away, and decided to have a quiet day, and look at them later, when perhaps I'd feel more like it.

I was glad to be feeling significantly better, and I'd thought that that would make me more cheerful, but I found that being able to do a little more made me want to do a lot more, so it didn't work quite like that!

Linda came to see me one morning, and we reminisced about our holidays in Italy over a coffee, which I'd actually had the strength to make! We talked of Sarah, who always sent her best wishes to Linda in her letters, and agreed that as soon as I was fit again, we'd have to go back to Conegliano or Stroncone or Caserta. Linda was very positive about Dino! She helped me believe more strongly that what would be would be, and as she'd come and stayed with me three times, and learnt Italian so she could speak with my friends, she knew a lot about my other life, and it was very helpful and consoling to talk with her!

Lizzie kindly visited the following week, also for a coffee which I was up to making, and we spent a delightful hour chatting, which now no longer made me feel too tired. It was wonderful! I could hear all about my little god-daughter's progress, and her older brother's, and look forward to getting to see more of them the following year.

Granny and I started going out for little rides in the car with my parents regularly, and Rusty came too! The journeys broke up the monotony of being in the house all day, but the vibration of the car made my lungs sore after about half an hour, so we didn't go far!

It was so much easier not to live for hours at a time in my mind now I could do more. I could begin to take more interest in the television programmes that I saw, instead of watching reluctantly as a means of helping pass the minutes, and if we had visitors or neighbours drop in, I could join them and have a short chat that made me feel more 'in touch' with the world at large in England again.

I still had phone calls from Italy, thankfully, even after all this time, and they and postcards and letters kept me in touch with what was happening. Then I got a surprise present from a group of my Benetton students through the post. How lovely! I carefully unwrapped it, and there was a beautiful black Benetton make-up bag, with one red handle, one blue one, a yellow trim round the bottom, and a bright green zip fastener. It was fantastic! Inside it was full of all types of make-up, wrapped originally in black cardboard, with the Benetton colours round the edge – bright pink and red lipsticks, powders, blushers, multicoloured eyeshadows, eyeliners, and a make-up brush. I couldn't believe it! And with the present was a lovely card, saying in English 'Studying and studying again, with no improvement but always thinking about you, from your best students' – and they'd all signed! And in some ways I could hardly bear to read their names, having felt I'd let them down so badly, leaving them in mid-course... and I wept!

That afternoon my parents took Granny and Rusty and I for a little drive to Bury St Edmunds. It was very busy, but proved an uplifting outing, and I loved passing by the imposing abbey gate, and the remains of the wall, picturing the crumbling ruins of the abbey stretching down to the small, slow-moving River Lark! We saw the gem of the Theatre Royal, and resolved to all go to a play next summer, if we could!

Then at the end of the month, we drove into Newmarket, and looked at the cheerful Christmas lights down the high street. There were lovely big decorations, rounded jolly Santa Clauses, swinging from long green, festive, holly covered ropes, across the road! We saw a string of finely tuned racehorses heading for their morning exercise, and we stopped the car and waited while they crossed the road right in front of us, much to our delight!

When we got back home to Ridlow, there was my first Christmas card on the mat! I opened it immediately, and it was from Giovanni. We'd hardly stayed in touch after we'd separated, but he wanted to wish me well, and a good year in 1991, back to good health! We hadn't seen each other for over a year, and it meant a great deal to me that he still cared.

I went to bed thinking about Giovanni. One day stood out particularly in my mind. We'd gone to his home town of Vittorio Veneto, and it had poured with rain. He'd told me that the people who came from the part of the town where he was born were nicknamed the radishes, by the locals! I couldn't remember why he'd said that was! We'd walked through the gracious part of the old town called Serravalle, and talked about our hopes and dreams and felt especially close that day.

Giovanni and I had left Vittorio Veneto in the early evening, and gone back to mine to make spaghetti alla Carbonara – with eggs and cheese and bacon. I'd happened to mention that I thought it was a marvellous dish, but that I'd never plucked up the courage to actually cook it! "No problem," Giovanni had immediately replied, "it's one of my specialities!" And so it had proved to be! Absolutely delicious!

Giovanni standing in Vittorio Veneto, under his umbrella, on that grey, gloomy day with the light rain pattering down, came back to me. He hadn't said much about himself on his Christmas card, and I wondered if he was happy. He was a good person, and he deserved to be. When he hadn't been busy, he'd very occasionally taken me out for a memorable day – to the Roman town of Aquilea, for example, and he'd got on well with Richard, better than Dino. Giovanni and I had had some good times together, without getting serious, and I was glad to have them come into my mind.

Chapter Twelve
December 1990

Andrea and James came round for tea at the beginning of December, and it was lovely to see them. They were going to spend Christmas with us, then go to James' parents for New Year. They were extremely happy in their new house in Ridlow, and James didn't mind his long drive to work. I found it easier to talk to them than it had been since the beginning of my illness, for my head was clearing, and my brain was not so muzzy.

Perhaps I would be able to get back to teaching by the summer of '91, as Linda and Lizzie thought! They were sure I'd get a job at my old school in Cambridge. In some ways it was an enticing prospect, for I'd loved the warm and friendly, supportive atmosphere from colleagues and students there, but... they both knew where my heart really lay now!

"Come on," I said to myself, "think about all the good things in Cambridge! You know you love it really!" And I forced my mind to tear itself away from Italy and think of the College Backs, the evening sun illuminating the front of King's College Chapel, so that it appeared a framed, glowing and exceptional façade among the trees, the wealth of well-stocked bookshops, the orderly Botanical Gardens, with their peaceful beauty, which I'd used to walk through each morning to go to work... Yes, Cambridge and its reality were returning slowly slowly to my mind.

I received a lovely Christmas card and letter from Richard, with some more bills for me to write an Italian cheque for, and learned that he was going home to Wales for Christmas. He very kindly offered to bring some of my personal things over to England in his car, in the summer, as he'd be driving home. I was extremely grateful, as I could certainly do with some more clothes!

My father came in with the shopping and put a heavenly smelling new wholemeal loaf down on the table! It took me straight back to Centurano in my mind, the little suburb of Caserta, where there was a bakery to be found by going under an aged archway, and across a square, dusty courtyard and through an open door at the far end. There, ranged in front of you were piles of flat, round, brown wholemeal loaves, dusted with flour, invariably having just been removed from the oven, and smelling divine! There'd be crusty apple tarts, too, and a matter-of-fact elderly lady who'd hobble over and tell you to help yourself before she'd take your money!

I got an early Christmas card from Maria and Sergio too, saying they were thinking of learning conversational English at the school where Richard taught, and coming over to see me in the summer. That was great!

There was plenty of room in the house for friends to come and stay, only I didn't want to put too much strain on my parents, as they had a lot to do with Granny, and my sister Andrea, and me. If I was up to entertaining, it would be a joy to have Maria and Sergio for truly as long as they liked, otherwise it might be wiser to stick to a couple of days. We'd have to see how things were, nearer the time!

Granny had started going "uh uh uh uh" to herself now, quietly under her breath, as she said it helped her to breathe better! It could be intensely aggravating, and sometimes we'd briefly take her off, to show her what it was like, but she took no notice and carried on! Instead of listening to her doing that all the time, I'd sometimes go into the dining room alone for the afternoon, willingly giving up the fire!

I thought about where I was living, in Ridlow, and what I related to most. I loved the country walks best. My brain was so addled... I couldn't think of much, but I jotted down the shortest and simplest of poems to help myself focus on the positive aspects of where I was living:

Autumn In Ridlow

Golden, russet, brown,
Scrunching through the leaves,
Hedgerows clipped back, sparse
Pheasant ducks and weaves

Rose-hips shiny red
Old Man's Beard dull white
Blackberries inky black
Sunshine faded, bright

Stubble mellow gold
Furrows all ploughed in
Fir cones on the ground
Conkers out to win

Green field freshly mown
Perfume on the breeze
Glimpse of All Saints' church
Nestling in the trees...

If I put my mind to it, I could also conjure up heart-warming scenes of Bury St Edmunds, walking round the enchanting Abbey Gardens, for example, and marvelling at how clever and effective the inspired planting was – or Felixstowe, where we'd been so thrilled to go as children, bracing ourselves against the wind when easing out from behind the windshield and having a cold dip before lunch!

One morning I had a very welcome card from my colleagues at the Linguistic Centre in Venice, with signatures all over it and, enclosed, a smashing letter from Cristina, telling me how the yearly courses had gone, especially the progress of some of my students. She also explained that she only had her thesis left to do before getting her degree! We'd all had such a good working relationship – seeing that sometimes one or other would bring in cakes for everyone at coffee time, now and again I'd taken some of my local Conegliano ones – or a selection from the bar near the university, so I didn't have to manoeuvre flimsy packets through the packed carriages on the train!

I also heard from the director of my English school in Caserta, and colleagues from the grammar school in Maddaloni, in the south, who had written to my Conegliano address, assuming I'd be well again by now, which Richard had kindly forwarded on for me. It was so lovely to sit down and open the envelopes, having guessed who they were from, and hear how they were getting on! I'd had two years in the south that I wouldn't have missed for the world! I'd never had a day's illness there, not even when one winter a horrendous flu was going round, and felling even the most robust! The climate had really agreed with me!

One afternoon Linda came round with a couple of her heavy albums of our holidays together, and we exchanged small Christmas gifts, and reminisced a bit more. I'd bought her tiny present, along with just about all the family's parcels through catalogues, to save someone having to go and choose things for me!

Lizzie also came that week to wish me happy Christmas, and warmly asked me to go and stay with her family for a weekend in Cambridge, as soon as I was well enough. I explained I was worried about upsetting her children, should I not feel good but she replied that I could go and rest when I liked, and that the children were very accepting, and wouldn't be put off at all!

As I went to bed and contemplated the New Year, I tried not to worry about it, and 'go with the flow'! I could hear again in my thoughts *The Last Post* being played in Caserta, as the wild dogs howled, and remembered how I'd loved the second year there, when we'd lived on the top floor of a modern block of flats, overlooking Caserta Vecchia, the old medieval town, on the hill. It was always a beautiful view, but especially so in springtime, with the peach trees in blossom below our windows, and all the plants bursting forth into new life. I'd often drive up alone to Caserta Vecchia, when Umberto was at work, for I felt completely safe there. I might see an elderly farmer walking slowly up the hill, with a pile of scrubby sticks balanced on his shoulder, or little children playing happily near the car park. I'd leave the car, and walk around the picturesque streets, sometimes popping into the lovely Romanesque cathedral, occasionally stopping for an ice cream lolly, and always looking down to the town below, which seemed to be covered in a blanket of haze, and I wondered if that was pollution.

That panoramic top-floor flat that Umberto and I had rented in Caserta had had a balcony all round, and French doors leading out onto it, instead of windows. Sometimes we didn't close the shutters at night, as no one could see in to us, and we'd awaken to the sun streaming through the French doors, even at that early hour warming the room, and see the old town illuminated, so beautiful on the hill.

It was strange to think how much I'd followed in my father's footsteps, by living unwittingly at first in some of the places he'd been posted to during the war. Caserta's Royal Palace, where he'd worked, was only nearby – and when one day there'd been a car bomb, damaging several cars near the barracks, I'd thought of him.

As Christmas approached, I had an urge to break out of my usual pattern of wearing hardly any jewellery, and put on some different earrings and a bracelet. I had in mind the gorgeous gold and sparkling earrings from my generous students at Benetton, and a very lovely bracelet from my extremely kind and also much-loved students at the Institute in Mestre. It had been a Christmas present last year. I'd taken some mince pies over for their last lesson, and very few people had been there, as so many had caught the bad recurring flu that had been going around. I'd been so surprised and delighted with my gift, and had never yet worn it. I'd missed my students too much to feel happy wearing it. Finally, after a year in Ridlow, I felt over the worst of the shock of leaving them so suddenly.

I took the bracelet out of its red cardboard box, and pale grey felt bag, which protected it! It was made of glass, edged and laced through with gold, with deep pink flowers and bottle-green leaves – two of my favourite colours. It glistened in the light, and looked almost too good to actually wear! I had never seen a similar bracelet before! As I put it on, I felt sheer joy!

My mother came in and I showed her, and she was most unimpressed! She said it wasn't her taste at all! It reminded her of India, she said, as though in a negative way. I loved it so much, like I did my beautiful Benetton make-up bag and earrings, because they weren't only beautiful in themselves, they made me feel close to the beautiful, thoughtful, kind students who'd bought them and so they warmed me inside.

As Christmas Day approached, I thought of the same time of year twelve months ago, and finishing off my courses for the holiday, so unsuspecting of what lay ahead... and of the last evening meal I had had out with Dino, before flying home to see my family. Maria and Sergio had recommended a wonderful place in the hills that was a little more costly than some restaurants, but where there was a special romantic atmosphere and a welcoming log fire – and the steak, which Dino liked a lot, was char-grilled and fantastically tender! I hadn't eaten any meat for over a fortnight, so I didn't feel guilty joining him. I just thought that as I'd been so busy of late, and sometimes more tired than usual when we'd gone out, it would be a good way of doing something that Dino would really enjoy, as a way of saying goodbye for the holiday!

Just as Maria and Sergio had indicated, the correct hill with the restaurant on had been a bit tricky to find! But how worth it it had been! The tables, exactly as described, had been covered in weighty red cotton tablecloths, with red cotton napkins, and the successfully placed wall lights had red shades, so there was a healthy glow to the room and each other's cheeks! We'd eaten simply, having well-done steak and mixed salad, and fresh fruit, with red wine instead of our usual prosecco. There'd been no high emotion, or outstanding news to report, it had been a comfortable, easygoing experience. On the other side of the room sat my accountant, with her husband, and an older couple, who looked as if they might have been his parents. We'd nodded and smiled to each other, and how good I'd had no inkling then that my world was about to change!

The next day, before taking me to the airport, Dino had given me my Christmas present. The previous year he hadn't given me one, as he hadn't wanted me to think he was interested in becoming too serious! I'd got him a walkman that last evening I saw him, so he could listen to his beloved football if he was out and about. And he'd given me a dainty gold necklace! His company had just completed the furnishing of the shop, and he'd seen one he knew I would like. It was encased in red felt with gold writing. A light, patterned chain became smooth at the front, either side of two clear-coloured stones, with a pale blue one drawing the eye to the middle. I decided to wear it for the first time on Christmas Day.

I had no photographs of Dino, and that necklace was the only tangible thing I had from him! I knew that whatever happened, it would always mean a lot to me, because we had been so in tune with each other when our presents had been exchanged.

I lay in bed again, looking round my bedroom, just as I had done when I had first got ill. I was interested to note that I could still remember my green bedroom in Conegliano exactly, and that I'd managed to imagine the glass chandelier and the painting over to Ridlow in my mind, as I'd hoped to be able to do a year ago, to soothe me slightly all this time! Perhaps if I was still ill next summer, Richard might be so kind as to bring the painting over with the clothes – by then I might have had to let everything go! It would take some doing without me there in person, but I accepted that it could well be a necessary step.

Even if I only got seventy per cent better – enough to go out and about and do a bit more, it would seem like heaven! I was weary of having these never-ending flu-like symptoms. My number one priority for 1991 was going to bed only at night – not needing to rest during the day!

We had a quiet family Christmas, and I stood up to it well, which was marvellous! I had no ill effects the following week. On the last day of the year, I spoke to Dino, and he agreed to come over in the summer, if I wasn't up to going back to Italy – for ten days. At least, one way or another, I was going to see him again!

My parents and Granny were more used to my illness, and we were more relaxed in each other's company. I was even used to eating in the evening by six o'clock! I knew that *they* knew I was enormously grateful for their kindly looking after me, and no longer felt duty bound to thank them all the time!

Most importantly, my ME was nowhere near as bad as it had been a year ago, and although my step forward was a small one, it nevertheless improved the quality of my life a great deal. I did the same things, reading a couple of short articles in the paper, having a chat, resting, but I didn't feel so *awful* while I was doing them! If only more energy would come back too. I still couldn't really count on any plans for the future, but at least I was less convinced that I was going to catch another terrible bout of flu, while my immune system was so weakened, and die.

Through having been given a chance to rest a lot, and using homeopathy, vitamin and mineral supplements, acupuncture, a plain and high protein diet, and praying quietly every day, perhaps even having Rusty to confide in, and friends' support, belief in myself, I'd got to know the inner me a great deal better than I had done when ME arrived! I'd had what sometimes seemed an almost endless year to look back over my past, and reach greater peace!

Now I wasn't finding that I restlessly flitted off to Italy with my thoughts all the time! I could choose whether or not I wanted to 'go' there. I could at last bear to face the fact that I was no more and no less than a very ill person in England, not a teacher any more, and not gadding about at all – for the time being!

Having more peace of mind from accepting my situation, and understanding my emotions towards Umberto and Dino better, was my greatest joy. I knew I should be able to face the future with confidence, if only I could! My previous lifestyle required a lot of energy, there was no denying it! Perhaps it *would* all come back, I reassured myself yet again!

In any case, I realised that over 1990, I'd laughed more than I'd actually cried, and that I'd managed to keep a sense of humour, even when I was shouting syllable by syllable something to Granny for the third time! I knew that I had to keep that love – of life, of people, and also love myself, for ME to be better endured!

I closed my eyes, and started drifting off to sleep, feeling very positive! Conegliano, I told myself, was in such a good position for getting out and about, to the sea, or to the hills, or the mountains, or picturesque small towns, or Venice at weekends, and to the rest of Italy on longer breaks! I persuaded myself that I'd get back and see it all again, and that until then my mind would hold the memories, and await the time they could be renewed! I was so much better! Ridlow was a good place too – there were the long, inviting, beautiful country walks around about, there was the proximity of Cambridge, Felixstowe, Bury St Edmunds, Colchester, Norwich, Newmarket... the excitement at the prospect of a sightseeing trip to London as soon as I got well enough! My spirits rose further. I was glad that I had come to terms with being in England! Dino might well come over and love it! I registered the fact that I was living with my thoughts in both countries now, which was so necessary if I were to be happy where I actually was. It was great to finally feel my thoughts had adjusted to having Italy no longer wholly dominating them, but allowing England, finally, to be *equally* – with Italy – on my mind.

Forthcoming Work

A later volume, *ME and Me* will detail how Anne Brewer worked towards full recovery from her illness, and achieved her goal of returning to Italy.